second opinion

second opinion

A STEP BY STEP HOLISTIC GUIDE TO
LOOK AND FEEL BETTER WITHOUT
DRUGS OR SURGERY

Rob J Smith

HOLISTIC EXERCISE THERAPIST

Ordering Information: Quantity sales. Special discounts are available on multiple purchases by corporations, associations, and others.

For details, contact the "Special Sales Department" at the address above.

Second Opinion, Rob J Smith --1st edition, 2017

www.evolveglobalpublishing.com

Book Layout: © 2017 Evolve Global Publishing

ISBN: 978-1-64136-644-1 (Paperback)

ISBN: 978-1-64136-645-8 (Hardcover)

ISBN-13: 978-1977755391 (Createspace)

ISBN-10: 1977755399 (Createspace)

ISBN: (Smashwords)

ASIN: B0721QJPGS (Amazon Kindle)

This book is available on Barnes & Noble, Kobo, Apple iBooks (digital)

Acknowledgements

I really need to acknowledge people that have had the most impact on my health, fitness and mindset philosophies.

Paul Chek, Pavel Tsatsouline, Charles Poloquin, Steve Denk, Troy Stende and Deanna Reiter, Dr. Freddy Ulan and Dr. Frank Springob, Eric Dalton and Dr. Eric Goodman

Mindset philosophy and spirituality: Earl Nightingale, Jim Rohn, Tony Robbins, Sonia Choquette and my life coach Julie Lyden who opened up a whole new life-changing world to me.

Special thanks to:

Our clients for always supporting my wife and me, our incredible staff that continues to get better every week and displays a level of professionalism, passion, and joy to help everybody around them.

My amazing assistant Jan Grundhauser who was with me every step of the way and ensured I got this book done and made it to best-seller status.

My illustrators and designers: Alex Turati, Arsyadi Yulian and Erwan Sulistiyo.

My daughter Sydney and her friend, Jenna, for helping me with the layout of my illustrations, and for always making me laugh, so I can spend more time with Dr. Happiness.

My biggest supporter and one of my greatest teachers, my wife, Paula. There have been countless times that she has led me in a direction that I needed to go in, spend time in and learn and master that area of my life, so I could help others. She has helped me get out of my head and start to trust my inner wisdom. She is an unbelievable holistic practitioner and life coach and she inspires me every day to get better!

Table of Contents

Introduction

The Doctor of the future will give no medicine, but will interest his patients in the care of the human frame, in diet, and in the cause and prevention of disease.

Thomas Edison

I want to start this book off by sharing the story of the person who actually inspired the title of this book.

Mike's Success Story

Mike was a 38-year-old professional that was experiencing constant and severe pain in one of his testicles, and it was starting to become debilitating. The pain was affecting his life tremendously, and he was at his wit's end.

He was in pain when he woke up, when he was standing, when he was seated and even lying in bed. He knew he had to go in and see a doctor, and then the first doctor he saw recommended he see a urologist.

They ran blood tests, they did an MRI, a CAT scan and they could find nothing that was creating his testicular pain. So ultimately the urologist said, "Well we can remove the testicle surgically, but there are no guarantees that it will take away your pain."

Mike swallowed hard and then politely declined the urologist's recommendation trying to process what he just heard. Mike continued to live with the pain. Trying to get some relief Mike was taking a handful of anti-inflammatory drugs every day.

A couple of weeks later he picked up the newspaper, something that he never does and there was an article about our wellness center, and he said to himself, "This sounds like exactly what I need, a holistic approach to my problem without drugs and surgery."

Mike first sat down with our wellness consultant Julie to go through his medical history. When she came back to me to explain what was going on, I didn't feel that there was anything that I could do from an orthopedic standpoint.

I thought he probably had a heavy metal or a bacteria or some toxin that was creating inflammation in his testicular region. I thought that it was something my wife would conclusively find by evaluating his nervous system. Using specific techniques, we can determine whether a symptom is caused by something nutritional, chemical, structural or even emotional.

I soon discovered through his evaluation that ultimately it was tight muscles that surrounded his pelvic region that was creating referral pain patterns. When I massaged around his hip area, I was able to decrease his pain by about 70% percent in just 15 minutes.

After my wife, Paula, did her evaluation of his nervous system she discovered he actually had some foods he was intolerant to which created inflammation in his body. This inflammation caused his deep spinal stabilizer muscles to shut down and in turn caused the muscles around his groin area and low back to get really tight because they were compensating.

His belly button, which is a scar, was also interfering with his deep stabilizing muscles working, so we treated it with a cold laser to deactivate the scar, and within three sessions he was completely pain-free. We went on to do two more sessions with fantastic results.

Obviously, he did not have to do surgery, was completely pain-free and functioning at a very high level. Sometimes you need a second opinion.

It also just goes to show you can't always judge a book by its cover and make assumptions like I initially did before I even assessed him.

What are the most important things in life to you? Typical answers people give are faith, family, friends, health, and my work. Based on what your answers are, can you say with conviction it is consistent with the time and energy you commit to it?

Anything in your life that is important, you will spend the time and energy investing in it. When it comes to your health, you're going to pay someone. You're going to pay the organic farmer, a holistic practitioner, a trainer, a gym, a supplement provider, a nutritionist, a pharmacy, a doctor or a therapist.

The difference is whether you want to be proactive or reactive with your health. Are you spending money on it or investing in it?

What is your plan for optimal health - do you have one? Or do you plan on just rolling the dice and letting your body take its course? Is your health something that is really important to you?

Your body is always changing, and it's either moving towards better health, or it's moving away from it. Most people tend to be reactive instead of proactive when it comes to their health.

Do you know what that means? They wait until they are somewhat incapacitated or at least very uncomfortable before they do anything to correct it.

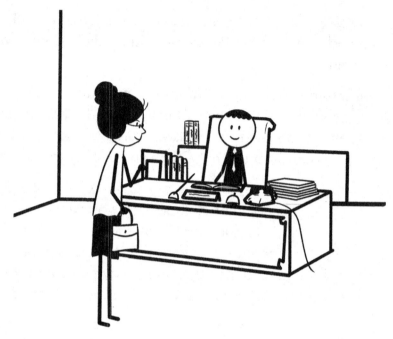

ALMOST EVERYTHING I HAVE HURTS AND WHAT DOESN'T
HURT DOESN'T WORK!

Today more than ever people are searching for alternatives to drugs and surgery. Conventional medicine really centers on these two options for whatever symptom you are experiencing.

Here is how it generally goes with traditional allopathic medicine. You have a symptom, they diagnose you, and then they prescribe. And you guessed it; the options are drugs, surgery and maybe some physical therapy.

Unfortunately, the conventional medical model isolates and compartmentalizes and only focuses on the symptom. Often times there are multiple variables that create a symptom. If you suppress your symptom, you will never get to the root cause of what is ailing you.

If the symptoms you are experiencing don't fall within specific parameters they can't diagnose, so many times they experiment with drugs to see if they will work on your symptoms.

Not long ago I went to a clinic to get my ears cleaned, and it seemed like the nurse just couldn't wrap her head around the fact I was not on any meds at my age. She kept asking me if I was sure I didn't have any other symptoms I wanted to discuss. I almost expected her to hand me a brochure with the title reading, Seven Simple Steps to Become a Hypochondriac.

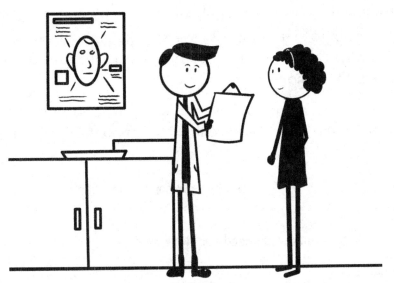

YOU'VE GOT A RARE CONDITION CALLED 'GOOD HEALTH'.
FRANKLY, WE'RE NOT SURE HOW TO TREAT IT.

Most people are very accepting of the diagnosis and prescription without questioning the doctor for possibly an alternative to a drug or surgical intervention, especially if their insurance covers it. Because people pay a lot of money for their health insurance they want to be able to use it and if something like alternative treatments isn't covered by their insurance, they are reluctant to move ahead with it, even if it feels right to them.

Have you ever received information from a doctor that just didn't feel right to you? I certainly did. That's a big part of what led me down the path to alternative health, and then on this crusade to show people there are options to drugs and surgery.

Conventional Medicine and Duct Tape

Even if you have tried multiple things that haven't worked for you, it's not too late. There is always a solution to the problem. Most physical conditions that people are treated for only address the symptoms.

If you take a drug or have surgery, you're not going to be getting to the real imbalance that is creating the symptom.

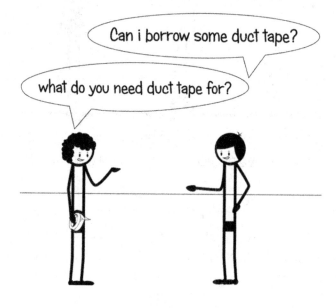

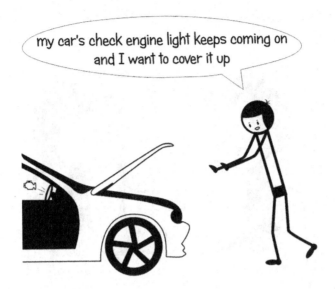

Your symptom is your body's way of communicating to you that something is wrong. Your body is telling you that you have an imbalance you need to fix. Our symptoms are brilliantly intelligent in waking us up if we are paying attention and understand this.

Your symptoms may be caused by a structural, nutritional, chemical, or even an emotional component that is stressing your nervous system.

But if you suppress that symptom, you will never ask a better question.

Most people ask, "What can I do to get rid of this symptom", instead of, "What is causing this symptom?" It's an entirely different mindset and one that can completely change your health picture. Symptoms don't just happen; there is a reason why they happen!

For some people to wake up, sometimes, they just need a wakeup call. True health is about the balance within.

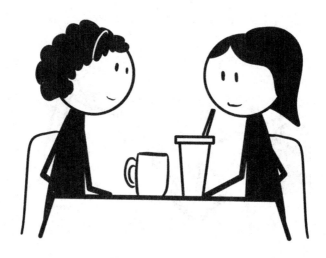

I DO WEIGHTS FOR MUSCLE HEALTH, CARDIO FOR HEART HEALTH AND CHOCOLATE FOR MENTAL HEALTH

Close your eyes and think back to high school biology, ah yes biology, and the term homeostasis. Don't you just get a warm fuzzy feeling thinking about it? It really is one of the most important things we can know about our bodies and one I will talk about in detail.

Our bodies need to have a balanced blood pressure, body temperature, muscle balance, ph balance and stable blood sugar or symptoms will show up, and bad things can happen.

Have you ever been very cold? What happens? Your body starts to shiver in an attempt to warm your body.

Have you ever had one of those really annoying paper cuts? Did you have to call the doctor? Of course not, your body went to work repairing your skin without any instructions from you.

What about breaking a bone? Have you or anyone you know ever broken a bone? What happens? The little bone repair factory inside you goes to work to fix the damage.

Everyone has a doctor in him or her; we just have to help it in its work. The natural healing force within each one of us is the greatest force in getting well.

Hippocrates

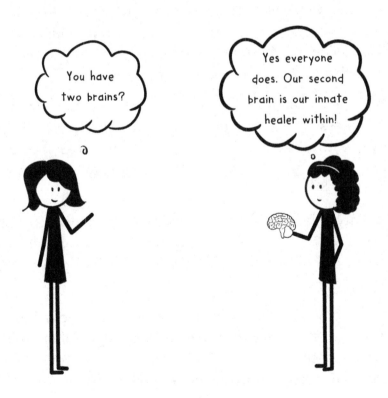

Everyone deserves to be healthy and express their full potential from the time they are born through their last breath of life. This includes you!

Our bodies have an innate intelligence to heal us from within provided we give it the best opportunity to do so. Present from the moment you were conceived, this intelligence guides the processes in your body.

Some of these processes turn the food you eat into cells, eliminate your waste products, coordinate your muscle contraction and communicate with or without your conscious thought via your nervous system.

As long as you have no interference to this system, you have the capability to heal, feel great, be healthy and function very well for a lifetime. Nurture this intelligence, and you will enjoy the health and fitness you were meant to have.

Your body can have interferences with the communication and expression of this intelligence. This interference in your body causes disease, disharmony, weakness, and imbalances within your nervous system. This can cause all types of immediate health problems.

Lifestyle interference is a result of poor health habits such as overeating, poor nutrition, excessive drinking, taking prescription or non-prescription drugs, or even sitting too much.

Environmental interference is caused by toxicity from air, food, water, or chemicals, as well as accidents. All three types of interference can cause interference within your nervous system and affect your health on every level.

The problem is when we start to get further and further out of balance. Today's science shows every organ in the body has the ability to heal itself. Every man and woman are the architects of their healing, sometimes they just need a little coaching, guidance, and support.

Just remember this, when we are in balance, good things happen in and to our body and when we are out of balance, bad things happen in and to our body.

Life is not a dress rehearsal, and we only get one body, so we have to take care of it, or we will be unable to do all the things we really want to do.

Life's Magic Moments

The older I get, the more my priorities change in regards to health, fitness, and aging.

Sure, I still want to look my best, but now it's become more about feeling good, moving well and about making sure I maintain the ability to not miss out on "Magic Moments".

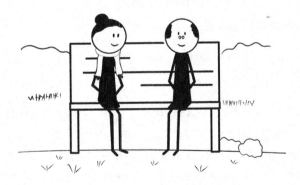

GROWING OLD IS LIKE BEING CONTINUALLY PUNISHED
FOR A CRIME YOU NEVER COMMITTED...

By all accounts, even for the most optimistic person, my life is half done, and I'm already feeling the urgency to do and see so many more things.

I would never want to miss out on any of these moments because I physically couldn't do something while others gushed with excitement over the experience. You may feel as I do that these "Magic Moments" are magnified when you experience them with others.

Maybe your magic moments are time with your kids or grandkids or your favorite hobby. My commitment to myself is to never miss out on the moments that are the most meaningful to me. Do you feel the same way?

One of my favorite movie lines came from the film, *Shawshank Redemption*, "Get busy living or get busy dying."

The ancient Egyptians had a beautiful belief about death. When their souls got to heaven, the gods asked them two questions. Their answers determined whether they were admitted or not.

1. Have you found joy in your life?
2. Has your life brought joy to others?

Good questions to reflect on. It is a lot harder to be joyful with yourself and others when you are sick and in pain.

My wife Paula and I feel so lucky that we've chosen a career in holistic health and fitness that has brought us so much joy. We never get tired of the stories our clients share with us about how different their lives are after going through our programs and the joy they are now able to experience.

Our Bumpy Road Led Us to a New Path

But our health journey has had many bumps in the road. We have had to endure so much suffering to get where we are today.

Our own health challenges have been allergies, hormone issues, digestive problems, blood sugar issues, chronic fatigue, depression, and chronic pain. My wife found herself at times crawling on the floor in the depths of her depression and feeling so burned out and hopeless because nobody could give her any solutions to her problems.

She was literally on death's doorstep because of her depression. She had a significant medical intervention without relief. Anti-depressants left her lifeless and fatigued. She was in a very dark place and felt alone, isolated and hopeless.

I had chronic pain on a daily basis, I struggled both physically and emotionally with the pain. When you have chronic pain and dysfunction, it is very draining on you. When you have health challenges, it can rob your energy, vitality, spirit and even your dignity. I went through the frustration of so many doctors and therapists telling me they had the solution to my problem, only to be disappointed time and time again.

I tried medication, injections, and surgery and none of them corrected the pain and dysfunction that I had from bone spurs and torn ligaments in my ankle, torn ligaments in my knee, shoulder, wrist and even a broken back. (I was in a brace from above my chest to the midpoint of my butt.)

My pain was so bad at one point with my ankle I almost felt like I could not endure it anymore; I would hop on one foot to get around the house to stay off my ankle.

It was a very daunting task just to do basic errands like go to the grocery store because it was so big and I dreaded the pain of walking through it. I would literally be lying on the grocery cart to take the weight off it to get some sort of relief.

The emotional pain of not being very physical and athletic was intense because it was part of my identity. I was also trying to hide the pain and dysfunction from my clients, because who would want to listen to the advice of someone who couldn't even "fix himself".

Even after two surgeries and multiple cortisone shots I still had chronic pain and reduced mobility, so I ended up seeing two separate orthopedic doctors to consult with about my options. Both told me because I was in so much pain, had insufficient mobility and could barely walk that a fusion of my ankle joint was probably the best option to correct the pain.

I wanted no part of that! Once a surgical procedure is done, there are no guarantees, and you can't get a do over.

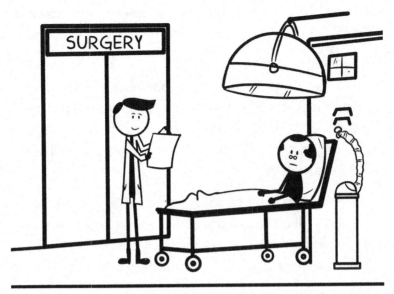

You have an 80% chance of surviving this and a 20% chance of wishing you hadn't.

Conventional medicine failed both Paula and me and led us to pursue alternative methods and ultimately to becoming holistic health practitioners. We continually seek to ask better questions as we work to understand the root cause of someone's health problem.

Most people's belief systems are shaped based on information you hear, see and of course your own life experiences. The definition of insanity, as many of you know, is doing the same things over and over and expecting a different result. We made a shift in mindset, philosophy, and lifestyle and it changed our lives.

My wife, Paula, and I are committed to sharing the message of alternatives to drugs and surgery to those that will listen. I am always intrigued by how people sometimes have opinions about health, therapy and fitness and they don't really know how they were formed.

When I ask them to tell me more about that, sometimes they realize that they didn't really put two different perspectives side by side and evaluate how they came to their conclusion. Maybe they got the info from their doctor, they read an article on it, or they saw it on TV.

Paula and I are very candid with clients, and we tell them we don't have all the answers, but over the years we have had literally hundreds of amazing stories of correcting client's pain and dysfunction and overall amazing body transformations when others couldn't help them.

People can refute our opinions or methods, but they can't deny our success stories. As they say, "the proof is in the pudding".

Pain and dysfunction are caused by a STRESS to your body, and it doesn't matter if it's emotional, nutritional or structural.

Remember it will always cost you time, money or energy regardless of what you pursue to fix your physical issues. The challenge is when that investment does not produce results because that's all people want, results to their problem! Isn't that what you would want?

When it comes to your health a better question to ask instead of how much does it cost would be, how much is it worth? Then determine if the investment is worth it based on the results it can produce.

Just because you don't currently have pain or a debilitating symptom doesn't necessarily mean you aren't out of balance. Your body can be stressed, but not stressed enough to create a response to get your attention. Eventually if not addressed, pain and dysfunction happen, and drugs and surgery are recommended.

The end result many times is just chasing your symptoms instead of getting to the root cause of your problem. Most people just don't know there are alternatives to drugs and surgery that can be much more effective.

You could even throw in conventional physical therapy because they only address the structural component to the pain. But many times there can be an emotional, chemical or nutritional component that is stressing your nervous system out and contributing/causing the pain.

Many times clients will tell me they did XYZ therapy and they "got better". But when I do their assessments I may find many imbalances that are causing the pain. So even though they no longer had pain when they finished their last treatment, they were never really "fixed" because all these muscle imbalances don't just show up, they've been there for a while.

When a therapist isolates where the pain is, and they just work that area, many times they will miss where the problem is actually stemming from.

I am always amazed talking with clients about the process they have gone through dealing with their condition. Typically, there is very little conversation with the client to gather information, as well as, in-depth analysis of the health challenge.

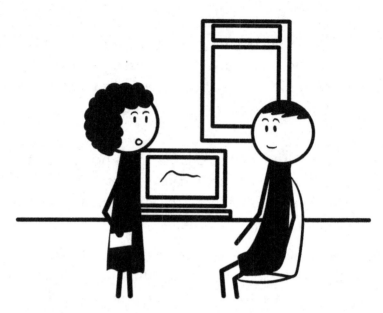

THE DOCTOR WILL BE IN SHORTLY TO TYPE ON THE COMPUTER
AND UPDATE YOUR CHART. IF HE HAS TIME, HE WILL ASK
HOW YOU'RE FEELING AND TAKE A LOOK AT YOUR RASH.

Over the years working with Division 1, Olympic and Professional athletes that had access to the "best doctors and trainers", they ended up coming to us because those "best doctors and trainers" were very good at isolating and compartmentalizing the issue but didn't get to the root cause. With this approach, too many people will just not get better.

Pro Athlete Success Story

In fact, one of these professional athletes we worked with had a food intolerance to eggs which he was eating every morning, as well as, an intolerance to wheat and they were causing inflammation in his gut. This caused his muscles that support and stabilize his spine to not work properly.

He also had an abdominal scar that was also contributing to his stabilizing muscles not working. We had to eliminate the things that were stressing out his nervous system and then teach his deep core muscles how to work the way they were supposed to, so they could do their job again, which is to stabilize his spine.

So working with all those doctors and trainers all they were doing was focusing on the symptoms. He would have never gotten better with their approach to injections, anti-inflammatory drugs, and exercises that were not targeting the correct muscles.

Our laboratory is our wellness center, and our clients provide physiological proof that these principles work and they work well.

Many of our clients when they came in to see us had already tried multiple doctors or therapists with little or no results and they were sick and tired of being sick and tired and in pain. For some of our clients, their pain is physical, for some their pain is emotional.

Belief, Hope, and Your Health

Sometimes you need more than a Second Opinion; you need belief and hope that you can get better. It seems most people have more faith in the fact that their disease, dysfunction or pain will win rather than the faith in the miracle that their body can recover, rebalance and rebuild.

Belief itself changes your biology; the power of belief is where it starts!

If someone wishes for good health, one must first ask oneself if he is ready to do away with the reasons for his illness. Only then is it possible to help him.

Hippocrates

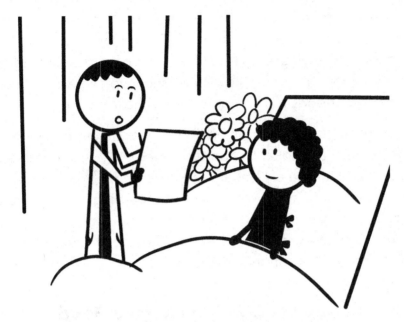

PLEASE DON'T PRAY FOR HEALING. IF IT WORKS,
YOUR INSURANCE WON'T KNOW WHO TO REIMBURSE
AND IT MESSES UP OUR ACCOUNTING SYSTEM.

When people come into our wellness center, they often become very inspired and hopeful when they see our dozens of success stories of people that found results with these principles when nothing else worked for them.

Although we believe most drugs and surgeries today are overprescribed and over performed, these are options that are available, and in the end, it is your body. Most people that we work with that have adopted our holistic approach were looking for a better and safer way to care for their bodies.

Based on my experience, **most** orthopedic surgeries performed today would not have needed to be performed. People are taking multiple drugs because one side effect from one causes another symptom and so on. What makes more sense, mask the problem, cut out the problem or determine what the underlying cause is? If you drug or cut, instead of correcting the imbalance, it will just show up somewhere else because your body will compensate for the imbalance.

I want to be very clear on one thing. If my family or I needed critical care at a hospital, the United States is where I would want us to receive that care. Lives are saved every day by the amazing advances in this part of medicine. But regarding getting to the root cause and uncovering the imbalances that create many of the physical issues people deal with daily, you're not going to get that from conventional medicine.

Our Health Stats Don't Look Very Good

People are aging faster today and not looking, feeling, or moving to their capabilities. The US spends about 14 million dollars per minute on what they call health care. Why do they call it health care? It sounds more like sick care, doesn't it?

We rank 11th to 37th in most statistical health categories. So we spend more than anyone in the world on health care, and we rank as low as 37th in some health categories like longevity, cancer, heart disease and diabetes.

7 out of 10 Americans take at least one drug. The average drugs taken by people ages 50 to 64 is 3.31, and I don't take any, which means someone's taking mine. The drugs taken by people of the age 65 to 74, is 4.45 and people ages 75+ are on 4.42.

People's bodies are breaking down so fast that they are having surgery done as if it was routine teeth cleaning. More and more people today suffer from depression, they can't sleep, they have fatigue, and digestive problems, allergies, joint pain, hormonal imbalances and they're aging prematurely.

In America today, we're usually told and believe that illnesses like cancer, arthritis, dementia, osteoporosis, diabetes, and heart diseases are diseases of the aging. But these chronic conditions are not the inevitable result of growing older, rather that they are the inevitable result of living a lifestyle that cannot support human health.

In America today, these conditions actually have reached epidemic proportions. And there are really no signs of these conditions slowing down.

As I'm sure you know, we are living in an information age and now more than ever you have access to anything you want to know about with just the click of a mouse.

We are drowning in information but starving for wisdom.

E.O. Wilson

People don't just want information, they want the truth! Big business is putting profits over people, and it's time to call them out.

Unfortunately, the truth can be hard to find with so many options out there. So much information out there has an agenda behind it. I recently saw a campaign with professional and Olympic athletes endorsing chocolate milk as the perfect recovery drink after exercise. Either they are completely selling out, or they are just that ignorant.

The commercial says, "Nutrients to refuel, protein to rebuild and it's backed by science". Even science can be bought and paid for and spun a certain way. Especially if it's paid for by an organization that has the money and resources to spin the science any way they want.

The book, *Milk the Deadly Poison* is a fantastic read that will give you the real truth about what I commonly refer to clients as "white pus" or if it's chocolate, "brown pus", other people call it milk. Do your own research, and you will quickly discover how bad it really is for you.

I am a truth seeker myself, and for most people, that's all they want, so they can finally get a solution to their problem instead of bouncing from doctor to doctor, therapist to therapist and facility to facility.

What's Your Strategy for Health and Fitness?

You can have all the motivation in the world, but if you are running east looking for a sunset, you'll never get there (right motivation, wrong strategy). It can be very disheartening when you put your faith in a doctor, a therapist or a particular program, follow it to the letter and don't get any results.

Wellness is inside us all, we just need to give our bodies the right environment, the right information, and the right raw materials to let it do its job. No matter how helpless you may feel, there is the answer to your health challenge, if you follow the right plan. But don't take my word for it, read some more amazing success stories from some of our incredible clients that have done just that.

I know these stories will amaze you as much as they have others and hopefully inspire you to take action so that you too can, "Look Better, Feel Better and Live Better, without Drugs or Surgery!"

My wife tells me sometimes I can be too "sciency", that's the technical term for using too much science to explain things, and I can be too serious at times. So I have worked hard with my three illustrators to create fun pictures, jokes, and analogies that people can connect with to make learning some of these concepts easier and a lot more fun.

I hope that you will find yourself smiling, nodding in agreement and maybe even laughing out loud.

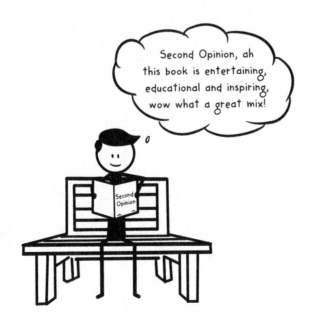

Chapter One

Stressors, Flow and Balance

What do you really need to do to achieve fantastic health and fitness while slowing down your body's aging process significantly?

What if you looked at your body holistically to get to the root cause of a symptom you were experiencing, instead of just suppressing it? Or what if you looked at your body as a system not just one part: but physically, emotionally and nutritionally. Would your health and fitness be different?

How in the world, with all the enormous advances in science and medicine, are we experiencing the largest epidemic of chronic diseases and orthopedic problems in human history?

I think most people are in physical bankruptcy because they don't know how to balance their bodies.

The further your body gets from optimal balance the more health challenges you will have.

Is your body in bankruptcy?

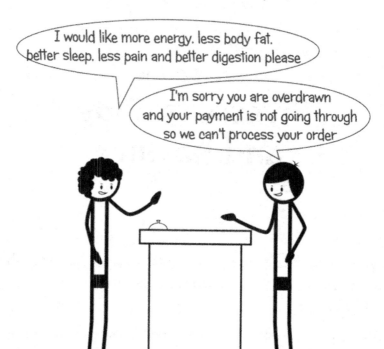

You know that if you keep withdrawing money out of your bank account without putting any back in, you eventually will be overdrawn. Your body works the same way. If you keep taking energy and vitality out and don't put any back in, you eventually end up in physical bankruptcy. So how do you fill your account?

Let's think of your body this way; a living bucket. Here is a list of stressors that will empty your bucket and can push you into physical bankruptcy.

Your Living Bucket

What empties your bucket accelerates aging and takes away from your health?

- Mental or Emotional Stress
  Negative thinking
  Negative people
  Bad relationships
  Poor work environment
  Worry

- Chemical Stress
  Personal care products
  New construction
  Pesticides
  Synthetic drugs
  Plastics
  Chlorine

- Immune Challenge
  Bacteria
  Virus
  Fungus
  Yeast

- Electro Magnetic Stress
  Microwave ovens
  Mobile phones
  TVs
  Computers

Electric alarm clock
Too much sun

- Physical / Structure
Poor posture
Too much exercise
Non-functional exercise
Muscle/ligament issues

- Nutrition
Eating: Too much, too little
Food intolerance
GMO foods
Artificial sweeteners
Trans Fatty Acids
Dairy

- Thermal
Your body being too cold or too hot

- Scars/Piercings
Episiotomy
Cesarean
Hysterectomy
Surgical
Belly button
Tattoo

Here is a list of things that that will fill your bucket, improve your health and vitality and keep you out of physical bankruptcy.

Your Living Bucket

What fills your bucket improves your health and slows the aging process?

- Meditation / Prayer / Deep Breathing
- Hydrogen Enriched Purified Water
- Sunshine
- Laughter
- Healthy relationships with Family / Friends
- Whole Food Supplements
- Organic Food
- Good Posture
- Stretching
- Tai Chi
- Chi Gong
- Restorative Yoga
- Walking
- Sound and Light Therapy
- Infrared Sauna / Infrared Mat
- Hobbies
- Following your core values

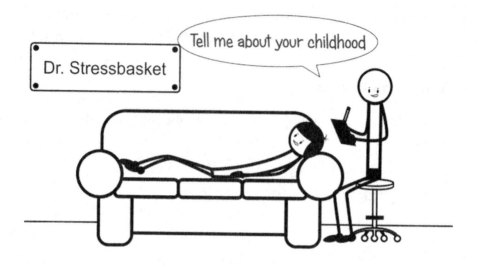

Stressors Are A Lot More Than Just Emotional!

Stress is what makes you sick and creates pain. However, when the average person thinks about stress they immediately think emotional stress. It's actually the stress response from all the external stressors that empties our buckets, not the stress.

When our bucket starts to empty it creates an imbalance and our body loses its capacity to handle the stress, so it shows up as a symptom. Our stressors are 24/7/365 days a year, so we need to have a strategy to fill our buckets on a regular basis.

Think of a stressor as anything that can knock your body out of homeostasis (balance).

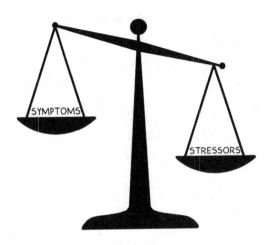

Disease and dysfunction are caused by an inverted way of eating, living, thinking and moving. Your internal body chemistry changes based on your nutrition, mindset, and lifestyle and you either move towards health or away from health. Balanced bodies are healthy bodies.

Some things you can control and some things you can't, but how you think, eat, sleep and move is under your control.

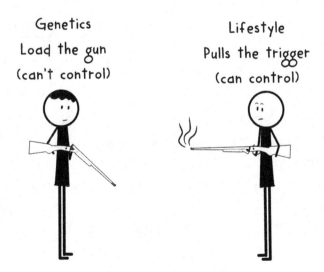

Your potential for super health and fitness can be described as harmony or balance within the body. This means your cells are functioning well and you have balance with your nervous system and muscles.

Speaking of your nervous system, let's understand it a little more. You have two separate divisions of your autonomic nervous system or as some people call it their automatic nervous system.

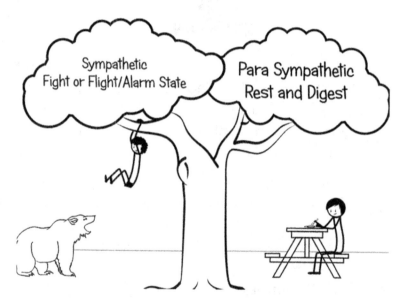

Think of living thousands of years ago as a hunter; you are going to activate your sympathetic nervous system (fight or flight) if you are either running towards your food as in hunting or running away from "being the food" as in being hunted. You managed to avoid being lunch and you were actually victorious in your own hunt and now you sit down to eat and your body switches to parasympathetic (rest and digest).

Your body needs a balance between these two branches, symptoms show up when you get out of balance. Your body puts on the brakes and you want to step on the gas or vice versa.

Today we do not have to run away from predators that eat us and most people just go to the grocery store or a restaurant for their food.

Your body, however, cannot differentiate between the stress of a wild animal wanting to eat you or stressors like chemicals, heavy metals, scars, tattoos, piercings, immune challenges or even emotional stress. Your body looks at stressors equally regardless of what the stress is.

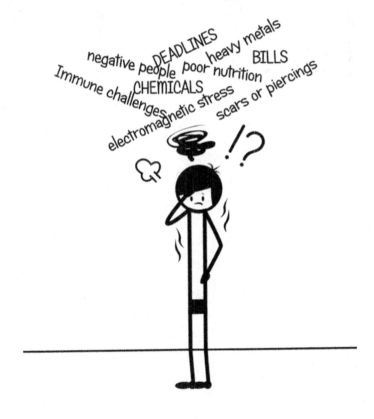

Because of all these stressors, most people are in an unhealthy balance of sympathetic dominance. Your body can not heal in a sympathetic state; it needs to be in a parasympathetic state to heal and repair.

Refer to your living bucket charts

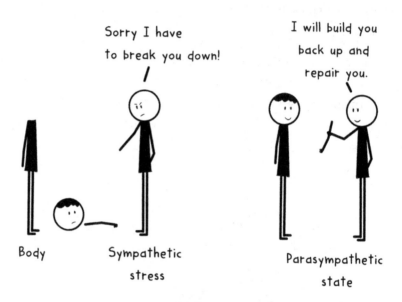

Joanie's Success Story

Joanie came to see my wife and me because as she put it, "My whole life and my body are a big train wreck". Joanie had irritable bowel, depression, low energy, chronic yeast infections, too much body fat and insomnia. When Joanie came in she said she needed some butt-kickin' workouts to try and deal with all of the stress in her life.

Joanie was going through a very stressful divorce, running three kids all over for school and sports, while trying to run her small business. She was struggling to cope with everything, so she would try to unwind with a couple glasses of wine each night. Joanie was very surprised when I told her I didn't think our group fitness training (boot camp) was currently appropriate for her.

She said after reading all of our amazing success stories, their results and how everyone said our group training was different from any other training they had done, she couldn't understand why I didn't think it was a good idea for her to start.

You see Joanie was in physical bankruptcy and intense exercise was the last thing that would be good for her. I recommended to her to focus on things that filled her bucket right now. Joanie needed to cultivate energy, not deplete it.

We supported Joanie's body with minimally processed whole foods and specific nutritional supplements that helped her get into a healing state (parasympathetic). We also taught her special breathing exercises along with using sound and light therapy to ensure we were rebalancing her body as quickly as possible.

In a little less than 90 days, Joanie got rid of all her symptoms and lost 34 lbs. without even exercising. Sometimes it's not what you're eating, but what's eating you that cause your body to become imbalanced. Joanie is now doing our personal training and has gone on to lose another 27 lbs. of body fat. Joanie was and

still is a very good student and now approaches her health holistically and proactively. Joanie says that her kids have never been healthier or happier because they got their mom back; a healthy, vibrant and fun mom sure beats, a cranky, tired miserable mom. Amen to that!

As I went through my training as a nutritional microscopist, (That's where I look at a person's live blood under the microscope; conventional medicine stains the blood and therefore changes the structure of it.) I studied the patterns of cellular health and imbalances that lead to symptoms and disease. I've learned that symptoms and eventually disease do not just randomly happen, it occurs for specific reasons.

Simply put, you need to put "good things" into your body and avoid having "bad things" enter your body. It is harder and harder to achieve optimal health because there are thousands more toxins today than there were 100 years ago. These toxins are in our water, food, air, personal care products, new cars and houses which include paints, stains, carpets and flooring and can potentially create health altering states.

We tell our clients that there are a lot of landmines they have to avoid out there while they are putting the good stuff in their bodies. There is also a lot of bad information out there that is confusing most people. Who do you believe? Who can you trust? Whoever you choose to work with, make sure they talk about restoring balance in your body. Your body is very unique and the stressors you deal with on a daily basis are different from anyone else's.

People who are truly healthy do not get sick. People that have good posture and good muscle balance rarely experience any joint pain unless, they experience trauma to that particular joint, but in general imbalances are the cause of joint pain.

Flow vs No Flow

When you have flow in your body, i.e....good blood flow, nerve flow and lymph flow, you have good health.

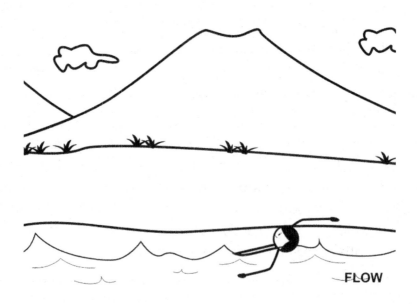

FLOW

Think of a beautiful mountain stream. There is vibrancy, there is powerful energy, and there is flow! I always feel amazing when I hike around a mountain stream because I can literally feel the energy and vibrancy that comes from it.

Another example of flow versus no flow is taking a bath or a shower. My wife is so relaxed she is almost sleeping after a bath, but is energized and full of ideas when she gets out of the shower. Start to think about flow versus no flow in your life. Healthy communication, ideas, goals, dreams, and happiness; let it flow!

When there's no flow, bad things happen in your body. What happens when you don't have blood flow to your fingers and toes? You have cold hands and feet. What happens when you don't have blood flow to your heart or brain? You have a heart attack or stroke.

When you don't have nerve flow, your muscles and organs are negatively affected and pain and dysfunction will occur. Eastern medicine refers to flow as life force, Chi or Prana. Western medicine talks about blockage. Blockage = no flow.

It is my opinion that this is where western medicine complicates things tremendously, this leads to confusion and fear and ultimately for most people treatments that include drugs and surgery.

Your lymph system is your body's second circulatory system. If you don't drain your swamp, i.e....move your lymph through proper breathing, exercise, massage, skin brushing or micro current, you will get sick!

Maintaining free flow of your lymphatic system is one of the most crucial elements to maintaining your health.

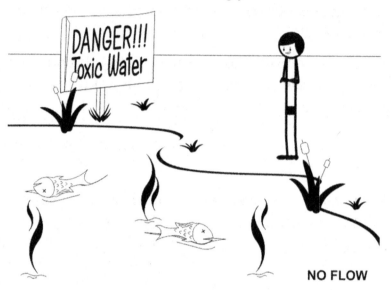

So what's the answer?

I don't think you need a doctor, I think you need four doctors. What? Hey, I'm not talking about the doctors wearing white lab coats with their stethoscopes hanging from their necks that are only interested in drugs or surgery; I am talking about the 4 doctors that live within us all.

The ancient Greek physician Hippocrates, also known as the father of medicine once said, "There are only 3 doctors that you'll ever need":

1. Doctor Diet
2. Doctor Quiet
3. Doctor Happiness

However, because of how sedentary people have become, one of my mentors, Paul Chek said, we also have to include doctor number four, Dr. Movement.

Spend more time with these doctors and I can assure you that you will spend less time with the doctors prescribing drugs and surgery. The principles in this book will allow you to, not only live longer, but allow you to enjoy a much higher quality of life, free of symptoms and disease.

Nobody wants to live a long time if they are in poor health and chronic pain. You want and deserve to be happy, healthy, vibrant and pain-free til the day you die.

You should want to have the physical strength and mobility to live your life on your terms. As you age you will either become a "classic or a clunker" You can only be one and you have the power to choose which one it is.

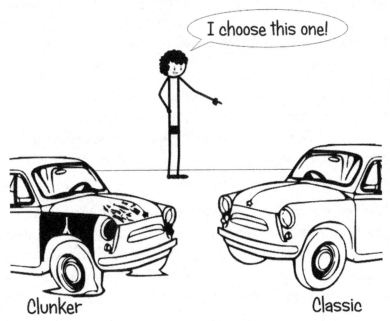

My wife will tell you that I am a very curious person and I love to people watch. I people watch at the supermarket, at the mall, at the local fair, when I'm hiking, when we are out to eat and my favorite is out on our patio watching the joggers. I'm always assessing how people are standing, how they are eating, how they are breathing, and how they are moving. I'll evaluate their posture, if they look happy, if they look sad, and if they look healthy?

I'm also a person who is very sensitive to energy. I love to be around positive people and I'm drained by negative people. I can feel people's energy without them saying anything and I will get out of a negative person's energy field as quickly as I can to protect my own energy.

Have you ever been with someone or talked with someone on the phone and when you are done talking with them you felt drained. Well, you are not imagining that. They are actually depleting your energy. If your energy field is healthy and your bucket is full, you can handle the stress load, but if your reserves are low, they will drain your life force or energy quickly.

Protect your mind as well as your body; negative relationships, negative news, negative self-talk, and gossip will all empty your bucket. There are times in life when others need to lean on us when they are going through a tough time, but always protect your own energy field.

The person with the weakest energy field will always draw energy from the stronger one. There is a very good reason a flight attendant tells us to make sure we secure our own oxygen mask before assisting others. Why? Because you can't help others the way they might really need if you are not at your best.

If your bucket is empty, you don't really have anything to give. The moral of the story, as my dad would say is, "Take care of yourself or you won't be able to take care of others!" And no you are not being selfish by making you a priority, you are being smart.

Better Questions Mean Better Health

Being a curious person by nature, I continue to strive to ask better questions with myself. I read something years ago by Tony Robbins that said, "The quality of questions we ask ourselves and others really determine the quality of our lives."

If you ask the wrong question, your self-conscious will work to give you a poor answer.

Let me give you an example. Some people will ask the question, "How come I can never lose weight?" Their brain will go to work and come up with really bad answers like, "because you never follow through, because you lack discipline, and because you hate to exercise".

A better question to ask would be, "What type of program will have me looking better, moving better, feeling better and enjoying the process?" Ask better questions and your brain will give you better answers and ultimately a better life.

Here is how my team and I approach certain questions when working with our clients. Instead of asking the question, how can this person get out of pain? We always want to know what imbalance created the pain in the first place.

If you are in pain you could certainly get a massage, take an anti-inflammatory, a pain pill or even have surgery to get out of pain. But the big question is, did you correct the underlying imbalance that created the pain in the first place? Or did you just eliminate your symptom? Isn't it time you got to the root cause of what's really ailing you?

For some people, it's a total mind shift from how they have been thinking. Does it make sense to you that when your body gets out of balance, a symptom will arise? Does it feel right to start listening to your body's signals? Not just listening, but actually trusting your body's signals.

My own journey has taken me from a 5th sensory person who was always in my head, looking for all the science and data to make a decision about my health, to now really listening to my own internal healer within. Whether you are familiar with and call it your internal healer, your 6th sense or just a gut feeling we all have it, unfortunately, most people just don't nurture it.

It's no different than nurturing a child, a pet or a plant; you nourish, they flourish. Nurture your 6th sensory self and it will reward you with better health and a better life.

Your mind can fool you, but your body never will because of the genius of our innate intelligence. Start to listen to your own signals and you will be surprised by what you learn.

I will find myself asking what I think of a certain situation and my wife will smile at me and ask me, "How do you FEEL about it?"

I can tell you without hesitation, I don't care how smart you are, you will never "outsmart your body"! Learn to embrace this gift you have inside you and you will forever be changed.

Chapter Two

Time to Assess Your Health

If you are like other people who come to us for help, then most likely:

You may have one or more health conditions that won't go away. You have visited allopathic doctors or even alternative practitioners, but the results weren't what you hoped or expected. You have health conditions that are significantly affecting your life. Perhaps this also affects your career, family, and/or personal finances. You realize that these conditions are probably not going to get better unless the real source of the problem is found and corrected.

Let's take a look at what a healthy person looks like:

High Energy * Clear Mind * Ideal Weight * Pain-Free

So what do you need to do to achieve optimal health?

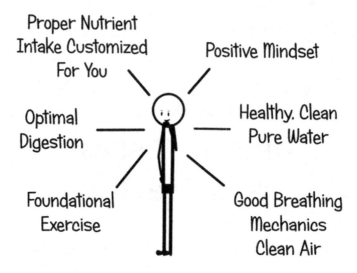

People often ask my wife and me if we can help them, a friend of theirs, a family member or even a co-worker with a particular problem they are having. We always tell them this, "If we're not assessing than we are guessing."

I don't know about you, but I don't want anyone guessing with my health. The first step when you are dealing with a symptom is to determine what is causing it. Doesn't that sound logical?

Any symptom can be caused by many different variables. Your friend, family member or co-worker could have the exact same symptom but caused by a different imbalance. If you don't get a thorough assessment, it is very difficult to develop a strong treatment plan. Cookie cutter programs frequently fail because the stressors that affect your health are different from others, just like your chemistry is unique to you.

The first thing we want to address is what exactly is stressing your body. Based on a combined forty plus years of clinical experience my wife and I developed a holistic chart that explains the stressors that affect your health by creating imbalances. Through a lot of trial and error and some very smart mentors, we created this system that restored our own health when others couldn't. We also use this chart as the foundation to heal all our clients that were not getting relief elsewhere. Start to think about your body as a system, not just individual parts.

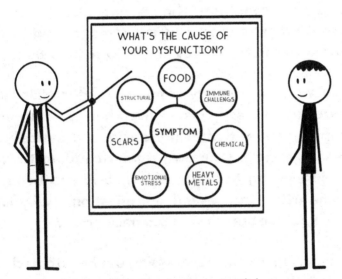

This Diagram that Rob and Paula Smith have created
Changed how people look at Health.
Health is not about treating symptoms,
but rather getting to the root cause

Stressors can affect your digestion, sleep, energy, joint pain, headaches, weight gain and your immune system. Every symptom is preceded by stress of some sort and your body's ability or capacity to handle that stress.

Haley's Success Story

Haley had many health issues when she came to us. She had so many digestive issues, and she bounced around to various doctors trying to fix her condition. The doctors she saw told her she wasn't producing any stomach acid and there was nothing they could do to help that.

My wife had a very simple fix after Haley's assessment, she just gave her a natural supplement of hydrochloric acid, and basically, it's the same as your own stomach acid. Instead of just giving her hydrochloric acid and being done with it, we asked the question, "Why is her body not producing stomach acid"?

She had many things stressing out her stomach; primarily it was foods and heavy metals.

As we went through this process, she needed less and less hydrochloric acid because we had addressed the root cause. Many holistic practitioners will use a basic symptom survey to determine what is needed, but if we hadn't found the stressors, she would have always just had to take a supplement. Instead, we helped her body rebalance so it could begin producing her own hydrochloric acid again.

She had the side benefit of losing over 20 pounds, and that's all she did!

Over the years we have focused on assessing our client's organs, glands, nervous system and their muscles so we could put together a treatment program based on what each individual tested for. We were able to produce great results with our clients, but we have always been looking for methods that are better, simpler and quicker to get results.

Cellular Health is the Key to Vibrant Health

If your body is comprised of trillions of cells, doesn't it make sense to go to the cellular level to solve your health problem instead of just suppressing whatever symptom you are experiencing?

Every plant and animal on earth is made up of cells, the smallest unit of life. Each of us is made up of about 75 trillion cells, and of course, not all of these cells are the same. We have over 200 different types of cells: nerve cells, blood cells, muscle cells, bone cells, etc. forming many different types of tissues.

This enables us to eat, breathe, feel, move, think and reproduce healthy cells which are highly resistant to disease and physical injury. Unhealthy cells create unhealthy tissues which are very susceptible to both disease and injury.

When you understand that pain and disease is a process rather than a thing to be cut out or suppressed, then you see why surgery and drugs are limited in what they can do and many times are just not the answer.

Cells can malfunction in a lot of ways, and the chemistry of these malfunctions can be very complex. All malfunctions can be reduced to two causes, deficiency and toxicity. Deficiency means your cells are lacking something that they need to function the way they are designed to function. Toxicity means that your cells are poisoned by something that inhibits proper function.

The cells in our bodies, in general, die for two reasons. First, because they did not get everything they need and second, because they get poisoned by something they definitely did not need. We can live long, healthy, vibrant lives if we do two things right: provide ourselves with all the nutrients our cells need and protect our cells from toxins.

Only after massive numbers of cells malfunction or die do you begin to notice symptoms of disease and pain.

When cells are not properly communicating with other cells, disease and dysfunction can occur.

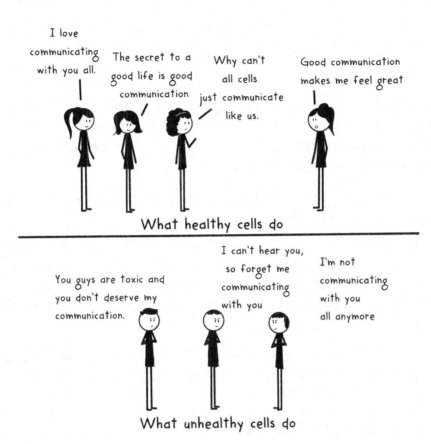

What healthy cells do

What unhealthy cells do

People who are truly healthy do not get sick. People who are truly balanced with their musculature do not typically have joint pain unless an injury occurred.

Illnesses do not come upon us out of the blue. They are developed from small daily sins against Nature. When enough sins have accumulated, illnesses will suddenly appear.

Hippocrates

Some people don't like to hear things like this because that means they are responsible for their health and not their doctor.

Over the past century or so dramatic changes in our diets, how our food is grown and our environment have created a society of nutritionally deficient and chemically toxic Americans. Sadly, the rest of the world is right behind us.

Virtually all of the foods we can buy at the grocery store are nutritionally inferior to the foods our ancestors consumed. The purity of the air and the water our ancestors enjoyed no longer exists. Fortunately, there are places where we can find good quality foods with high nutritional content, and we can certainly lower our daily toxic exposure. It all starts with learning how to take charge of our own health.

It is a daily battle to be healthy, vibrant and energetic, but it can be done. Your health actually begins at your cellular level.

Everything is Energy

Everybody that paid a little bit of attention in high school has heard of quantum physics, but very few people understand it or question it. Quantum physics has been accepted by the scientific community for more than 100 years, yet very little quantum science has been used in conventional health care.

Some uses are medical diagnostic equipment such as MRI's, CT and PET scans (An imaging test that allows the doctor to check for diseases in your body. The scan uses a special dye that has radioactive tracers. These tracers are injected into a vein in your arm, this helps doctors to see how well your organs and tissues are working.)

Alright back to the explanation of what quantum physics is; ok let's keep this simple, remember I promised my wife.

The science of quantum physics exists to explain the makings of the smallest pieces of a structure known to man. Your body consists of many "health systems", such as your digestive system, your nervous system, your circulatory system, etc. Each of these systems is made up of your organs.

Your organs are then made up of tissues, which are made up of cells. If you go even smaller, you discover molecules, atoms and sub-atomic particles, which are made up of packets of energy known as the "quantum" and everything in our universe is energy.

Did you know everything vibrates?

This Universal Law states that everything in the Universe moves and vibrates and everything is vibrating at one speed or another. Nothing rests; everything you see around you is vibrating at one frequency or another and so are you.

However your body's frequency is different from other things in the universe, so it seems like you are separated from what you see around you; people, animals, plants, trees and so on. BUT you are not separated, you are in fact living in an ocean of energy - we all are. We are all connected at the lowest level, and it is called the unified field.

The Law of Vibration

Everything has its own vibrational frequency; your table, your car, a picture frame, a rock, even your thoughts, and feelings. It is all governed by The Law of Vibration.

A table may look solid and still, but within the table are millions of millions of super tiny particles "running around" and "popping" with energy. The table is pure energy and movement. Everything in this universe has its own vibrational frequency. However since we can't see the energy, the table appears separate and solid to us.

The Law of Vibration is real, just because you can't see it does not mean that it is not true. We tend to live by the old saying "seeing is believing", so we should learn from history and realize that something might be true even though we do not see it. We do not have to see something to believe it, right?

Here are some examples off the top of my head:

- Gravity (we all believe it exists, but we can't see it)
- Cell Phones (we can't see the energy that allows it to work, but believe it)
- The Internet (we can't see the energy that allows it to work, but believe it)
- A Radio (we can't see the energy that allows it to work, but believe it)
- A Dog Whistle (science has shown dogs can hear sounds we can't)

Imagine having a conversation with your grandparents telling them someday we are going to be able to carry a tiny gadget in our pockets with the capacity to store thousands of songs, take pictures and enable us to talk to someone on the other side of the planet with no wires. As much as they loved you, they would have probably thought of taking you straight to the "loony bin".

But today smart phones with all these features are as common as fruits and veggies to many people all over the globe.

So how does this all relate to your health? Think of your body as a big giant battery of energy, certain things will drain us, and other things will recharge us.

Morphogenic Field Testing

The Morphogenic Field is a term we use to describe the field of energy around your body. The larger your energy field is, the healthier you are and the smaller it is, the less healthy you are. That makes sense, doesn't it?

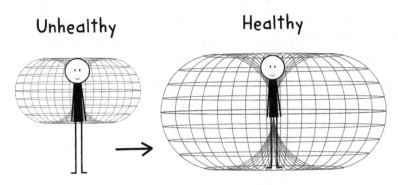

Your field is an extension of the electrical energy of your nervous system. Just as all electrical systems have electromagnetic fields that surround them; your brain is an electrical generator with its own field of energy that extends away from your physical body. Many cultures recognize this field and give it other names. When people discuss auras, chakras, life force or chi, they are possibly talking about this same energy field.

Morphogenic Field was named for this nutritional and energetic healing technique for a number of reasons. The word can be broken down into "morph", meaning "to change" and "genic" meaning "to originate". This is the exact goal in dealing with any health issue, and we use these energy fields to "originate change" in our client's health status. After we test our clients we then simply supply the nutrients they need to feed their bodies at the cellular level. This technique was developed by a brilliant doctor named Frank Springob and his colleague Autumn Smith.

During our evaluations, we rely heavily on information from the energy field of their cells to guide us in developing nutritional protocols for their unique needs.

Cellular communication is the ultimate goal. When we address the exact nutritional needs at the cell level, we affect the greatest change in a person's health. Remember, healthy cells are required for healthy tissues. Healthy tissues are required for healthy organs. Healthy organs then result in a healthy and vibrant body.

Kathy's Success Story

For most of my life, I have had stomach issues and chronic heartburn. I had seen many doctors over the years for this and usually walked away with a prescription for Prilosec. Obviously, this was not the solution I was looking for and sought help from Rob and his wife Paula to get to the root of the problem. Through the Morphogenic Field Testing, it was determined that I had wheat sensitivities and sugar issues.

After altering my diet and taking the whole food supplement recommended, my heartburn was gone, and the majority of my stomach problems disappeared. I also began having shoulder pain several years ago, but initially ignored it. As the pain increased, I began seeing a chiropractor regularly, had massage therapy and finally consulted an orthopedic doctor, who gave me therapy exercises and suggested cortisone shots.

I did not want to do the shots, and the exercises did not help. Nothing was working, and it continued to worsen and limit my mobility. I saw Rob, and one of his therapists Nik for therapy and my shoulder improved dramatically. I have not had therapy on that shoulder for 1 ½ years, and I still have full mobility and no pain.

My experience with Rob and Paula and their holistic principles have been life-changing for me. I will continue to share these principles that have so positively affected me with anyone that will listen.

"The energy field is the thing."

Albert Einstein

MFT is a foundational and clinical nutrition technique with an emphasis on:

1. Your body's innate intelligence
2. Your unique biochemistry
3. Addressing the issues with our modern diet and its deficiencies.
4. Recognizing how stressors are affecting your health
5. Customizing a very specific and customized program based on your body's imbalances.

Optimal Health and Energy Signature Matching

What does it mean to match the energy signature of your body to the energy signature of your food?

Your energy signature is greatly influenced by your immediate environment. What you eat, your level of emotional stress, toxins that have entered your system and hundreds of other factors including your genetic makeup all affect your energy field. In other words, your energy signature today is different from what it was last year, last week and even yesterday.

Your energy field varies based on your diet, sleep, stress and toxic exposure. Your genetics are the constant that doesn't change, but the variables, i.e. your stressors are always changing, this is why for optimal health you should regularly be assessed by a skilled practitioner. We recommend being assessed monthly to ensure your body is functioning at its best.

Your energy is represented by a field that constantly surrounds your body in a recognizable pattern call the "torus". In our work, we call this the Morphogenic Field or M-Field. In a healthy person, it is a large and balanced field that radiates off the body to approximately 5-7 feet, based on the MFT method of measurement. People with a large M-field are usually healthy, vibrant individuals. People with a small or distorted M-Field usually have some level of health challenge and are lacking in personal energy.

This torus pattern is found consistently in all forms of matter, from humans to planets and even galaxies. Food also has an

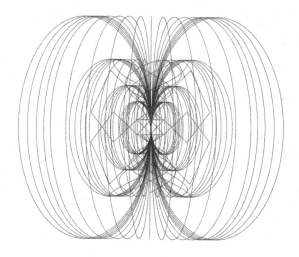

energy signature. The same torus pattern can be seen in the cross-section of an apple or an orange as in this picture.

In MFT, we consider the torus to represent the energy signature of the atom, the fruit, the human or the planet. We use this in combination with the science of muscle response testing to match-up the energy signature of food with the energy signature of the person.

In 1915 a man by the name of W.R. Lovett published the first peer reviewed paper on manual muscle testing in *The Journal of The American Medical Association* (JAMA).

The premise: Proper nerve flow will make a muscle stronger than partial nerve flow.

Nerve Supply and Your Cellular Health

Quantity- Improved with Chiropractic adjustments and other mechanical techniques

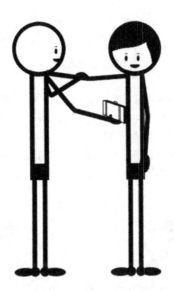

Energy Signature Matching Using MFT

Quality- Improved with optimal nutrition based on your needs.

Food is presented to a person's energy field with the intention of learning whether or not the food is an M-Field Signature Match to that person. If it matches, this food can be considered acceptable to that person. If the body rejects the food; we conclude that this food will not provide the body with the nutrients that it needs at that given time.

We have found that "matched food" is nourishing to the body and "mismatched food" is a stress to that person's body and can affect their health and well-being. I'm sure you can remember a time when you ate something, and you didn't feel very good after. If you consistently experience the same negative responses, you know you have probably proven this food, and your body is not a good match.

Our purpose in presenting this concept is to educate and empower people to seek food sources that will expand their M-Field so they can become healthier and more vibrant. If consumers demanded food that nourishes and fuels the body, it would go a long way toward developing a supply-and-demand situation that benefits our health instead of challenges it.

What if we could ensure the people who grew our food moved away from their current trend of degrading our food supply with processed and genetically engineered products? It's all about supply and demand; the more we demand healthier food, the more they will have to change their ways.

M-Field Signature Matching consistently reveals that only the energy of organic whole food truly matches the energy signature of the body. Something worth noting; we have never tested anyone positively for any food that was genetically modified.

My Road Trip Story with My Wife

Recently my wife and I went on a road trip and stopped to gas up along the way. After gassing up, we went into the gas station to get some sunflower seeds. Well, my wife is just as fanatical about her work as I am mine and she said, "Hey let's signature match these sunflower seeds and see if your body wants them."

All I could think about was that I wanted them, and I may have to use my special mental powers to make sure I tested positive for them. Paula tested me for the first brand, and my muscle immediately went weak, then she tested the second, same outcome. Yikes! Looks like Superman has found some kryptonite she said with a grin. I was bracing myself for the disappointment of not getting my sunflower seeds. She tested me with the third brand and what do you know, the third time was a charm.

What the heck was the difference we wondered? Paula turned around the package of the seeds I tested for and on the back of the package it said, Non-GMO Seeds. Sure enough, the other brands were genetically modified seeds. I avoided another landmine thanks to my wife, and it proved once again our bodies want food that nourishes us, not poisons us.

Karen's Success Story

Karen was referred to us from her chiropractor because she had chronic back and hip pain even though she was holding her chiropractic adjustments. After assessing her, we discovered she had a tattoo on her back right where the pain was. I mentioned to her tattoos and piercings can sometimes disrupt a person's nervous system and shut the deep core muscles down so then there is nothing to stabilize the spine.

She gasped when I said that and then told me she had 10 years ago had a belly button piercing and that's exactly when her pain started. It was enough to shut those muscles down and then because she never re-educated them to work the way they were supposed to, dysfunction started, followed by pain for 10 years despite working with multiple doctors and therapists.

She had just given birth to a baby girl; she was nursing and thought she needed extra calcium, so she was drinking more milk. After testing her, we found out that she was intolerant to milk as well as sugar. The milk and sugar were stressing her nervous system and created inflammation, so she got off milk and sugar, took the supplements we recommended and within two days her hip pain went away.

If Karen had only done physical therapy, she would have never gotten better. She needed a holistic model that didn't just focus on her structure. Very rarely is it just one thing that is creating pain or dysfunction that's why cookie-cutter programs won't work for a lot of people.

Lynn's Success Story

Lynn who was experiencing severe vertigo and she had struggled with it off and on for a little over three years. She had met with several specialists, and they tried several different techniques and medications with her and nothing was getting better.

Lynn was referred to us by one of her co-workers who is one of our clients, and we did MFT with her. We immediately identified that she had severe heavy metal toxicity. Lynn had some mercury fillings in her teeth that that were leaking and they were literally poisoning her body. After Paula identified the teeth that were leaking, we referred Lynn to a holistic dentist to remove the two amalgam fillings that were creating the problem. We also put her on a detoxification protocol to get rid of the heavy metals in her body. Her vertigo disappeared in just a couple of weeks and never returned.

Mercury has been evaluated and tested as the most poisonous metal to the human body by several studies. The most common places to get high levels of mercury are fish that are farm raised and from dental work, but you won't hear that from the American Dental Association.

I had the good fortune to interview the pioneer and probably the foremost expert on holistic dentistry Dr. Hal Huggins for a radio show I used to host. He wrote a fascinating book called; *It's All in Your Head*. I could not believe the damage mercury could cause to the human body and how this information has been hidden from the public. One of the many landmines most people will never know about.

MFT allows us to get to the root cause of a problem fast and put together a nutritional treatment program based on each person's individual needs. We work with the innate intelligence of each person's body. Your body can heal itself as long as you remove the poisons and feed your cells the **right** nutrition for you. Don't rely on some cookie cutter solution or you may never find optimal health.

Make sure whatever form of testing and health program you are on, that it is customized for your current needs based on all the variables that affect your health.

Chapter Three

Dr. Diet, Nutrition, Calories and Chemistry

Hippocrates once said, "Let food be your medicine and medicine be your food." It's important for most people to look at food differently than they might be currently. Why? Because as you will soon learn, it is how food affects your body chemistry that is important.

Think chemistry over math when it comes to how food makes you feel and positively changes your health. How food affects you is based on many different factors and your body is not going to respond the same as maybe others around you because of your unique biochemistry.

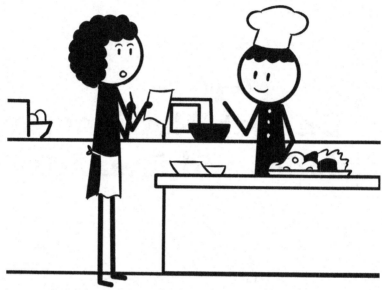

THE PODIATRIST WANTS JAM ON HIS TOAST, THE PSYCHIATRIST
WANTS NUTS ON HIS CEREAL, THE PLASTIC SURGEON WANTS
NO WRINKLES ON HER BACON, AND THE FERTILITY DOCTOR
WANTS HIS EGGS FROZEN.

Chef Luke

When I was younger one of my favorite movies was *Willy Wonka and the Chocolate Factory.*

Why? Because I loved candy! Although I did not ever get my hands on the everlasting gobstopper, it was like I did, because I was always eating candy. My friends and I would go do an odd job or two, get some money and then go right to the candy store. My paper route money went to two things, video games and sugar.

Thank God those two things didn't turn me into a gambling degenerate and a heroin addict. Studies have actually proven

74

sugar is as addictive as heroin. When I was in seventh grade, I was the ADHD poster child.

My poor mom would go to my school conferences and literally come home in tears because she had to listen to the teachers complain about how distracted and disruptive I was. I was also sick a lot, getting strep throat every winter and of course, we thought it was because I was playing hockey in a cold, damp arena. Mm hmm. Or was it probably just the truckload of sugar I was eating every day.

Did you know one tablespoon of sugar can suppress your immune system for five to six hours? Gee, I wonder if the reason illness increases during the holiday season has anything to do with the massive sugar consumption? According to my chiropractic friends their patients aren't holding their adjustments during the holidays as well either, possible connection to sugar?

Nah, I'm sure it's instead that all the bad bugs are just waiting to invade and attack our bodies during the holiday season and that's how we get sick, Ya know like Louis Pasteur's germ theory.

The Germ Theory and the Homeostasis Theory

In the late 1800s in France, the seeds were sown for two approaches to health—Germ Theory and Homeostasis Theory. Let's look at the Germ Theory first. Medical researcher, Louis Pasteur, made a momentous discovery when he discovered the existence of germs and that germs were associated with infections and disease. Many experts will tell you that others had already beaten him to the theory, but it was Pasteur who popularized it.

As a result, it became accepted that germs were the cause of infectious diseases. At the time Pasteur believed that the body was germ-free in its natural environment. The Germ Theory, even today, is still the accepted science by the medical establishment. The second approach to health was put forth by Antoine Bechamp and Claude Bernard. They suggested the Homeostasis Theory for health but did recognize the existence of germs.

Their message, however, was that germs are always with us and within us. These germs, they explained, only multiply to the point they create problems or disease when our internal environment is weak. In other words, our body processes or our immune system needs to be strong enough to keep the germs in check. The Germ Theory focused on killing germs to avoid or get rid of the disease. The Homeostasis Theory focused on strengthening the immune system to stay healthy.

What most people don't know is when he was dying Pasteur actually changed his view and agreed with Antoine Bechamp and Claude Bernard. Bechamp and Bernard said we get sick because of the way we eat, think and live; these things change our internal chemistry which weakens our immune system, and that's why we get sick. But heck there is no money to be made with that theory, after all, what would happen to all the drugs if that was really the case. (please note the tone of sarcasm)

On his deathbed Pasteur had completely changed his views stating the germ is nothing, the terrain (a person's internal chemistry) is everything. Of course, it fell on deaf ears because conventional medicine as we know it today already started that money train and there was no way they were going to stop it even if the man who popularized the germ theory to the world said it is not accurate.

I can tell you that I have personally had the flu one time in the last 20 plus years and I am always around people that are sick. Not sure how conventional medicine would explain that based on the germ theory. Maybe the germs just don't have my address. I also very rarely ever get a bad cold and when I do it might last a day or two, but often I will go a couple of years without one.

Are You Tending Your Garden?

There is a specific ratio of good and bad bacteria, i.e... Good bugs and bad bugs you need in your body at any one time. When bad bacteria increase in your body, your immune system becomes weakened and overwhelmed.

Ever get the feeling you're not alone? Maybe it's because you're not. Your body is a walking hotel for microorganisms, and their cells outnumber yours 10 to 1. Some of us have herds of mites grazing on our eyebrows. Others have fungi hanging out between our toes, I know kinda gross. No one is immune. Everyone's skin swarms with an invisible buffet of bacteria, and our mouth is a microbial wonderland. But it's the 500 or so species of bacteria residing in our gut that really make us tick.

Yes, bacteria account for a large majority of the 100 trillion creepy crawlies that call your body home, and they flourish in the dark, moist folds of your GI tract. (Random parasites, yeast, and fungi make up a much smaller internal population.)

Good bacteria spend their days destroying their harmful cousins, picking through undigested leftovers. But when stress, alcohol, medications or a poor diet (among other factors) lay waste to these friendly bacteria, bad bacteria rush in to fill the gap. When bad bacteria prevail, illness strikes. A short-term imbalance can lead to diarrhea, bloating and gas. Over time, the imbalance can contribute to more severe problems, including inflammatory bowel disease and irritable bowel syndrome.

Think of your insides like the soil of a healthy and beautiful garden for a moment.

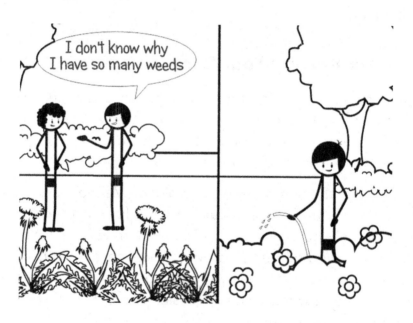

If you don't tend your garden, the weeds will overtake your garden. The weeds are like bad bacteria, and they will come and take control of your insides. If you are sick, it's because you have not been taking care of your garden's soil. The first step in growing healthy and strong plants is to start with good, healthy soil. That's how organic farming is done, and the same principles to growing healthy plants will help us have healthier bodies.

Is Big Corporate Farming Putting Money over Our Health

According to the Nutrition Security Institute (www.nutrition security.org), U.S. soil is eroding 10 times faster than it can be replenished. Researchers who compiled reports from around the world conclude that U.S. agricultural soil has been depleted of 85 percent of its minerals and vitamins during the last 100 years.

Other parts of the world report similar or worse soil conditions. In 1914, the report says, there was 400 mg of (sums of averages) of calcium, magnesium, and iron in U.S. cabbage, lettuce, tomatoes, and spinach. In 1997 (the last year figures were available), that mineral content had shrunk to 75 mg. Head researcher Don Davis, of the University of Texas Austin's Department of Chemistry and Biochemistry, says that modern agriculture's focus has been on size, growth rate and pest resistance, not the nutritional content of the plants produced.

The plants, unable to keep up with growth, cannot manufacture and fully uptake soil nutrients. You can't have healthy plants without healthy soil. This is one reason why organic food is better, it has more nutrition and no toxins, and that's how nature intended it to work.

Big farming operations rely on chemicals to maximize yield, but back in the day farmers like my grandpa used manure spreaders to help produce healthy soil. Both of my grandparents were farmers, and it was like a beautiful symphony watching nature the way it was intended to be. On their farm you would find uncaged chickens pecking away for food, cattle grazing on plentiful grass, grandma in her amazing garden growing strong, chemical free and nutrient rich food and grandpa on the tractor spreading that magical manure.

Animal manure, such as chicken manure and cow dung, has been used for centuries as a fertilizer for farming. It can improve the soil structure so that the soil holds more nutrients and water, and therefore becomes more fertile. Animal manure also encourages soil microbial activity which promotes the soil's trace mineral supply, improving plant nutrition.

Today we have whole industries created because of Pasteur's germ theory, that in the end, he didn't even agree with.

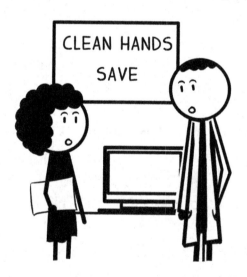

I USE SO MUCH ALCOHOL-BASED HAND SANITIZER,
MY HANDS HAD TO JOIN A 12-STEP PROGRAM!

Don't think hand sanitizer; think about healthy soil and a healthy garden! A drug suppresses symptoms, and with a healthy internal soil, you have no symptoms. As a nutritional microscopist I would look at people's blood under the microscope at very high magnification and the worse their symptoms were, the worse their blood looked. People were fascinated by the comparisons of what their blood looked like (their soil) and what a healthy blood picture should look like.

When I was young, I certainly did not take care of my internal soil that's why I was sick so much. I would have probably been obese, but exercise was my saving grace. I was moving from sun up to sundown in the summer time. You're probably thinking with all that exercise at least I probably drank a lot of water.

For optimal health a person should drink half their body weight in ounces of pure filtered water, so a 200 lb. man, should consume 100 ounces. For the most part, the only clear liquid I was drinking was, wait for it, 7-Up!

Of course, I drank water, but it usually had Kool-Aid or lemonade mixed in it. Yes I know now it is horrible, but I was too addicted to sugar back then to really care.

And things weren't getting better on the nutritional front as I got older. My sophomore year in high school my girlfriend was a waitress at a local restaurant, and when she got off work, she would go to the store and get me my three favorite things at that time, a six pack of Mountain Dew, a one pound bag of red Twizzlers licorice and a half gallon of butter brickle ice cream.

During a movie and I would polish off two Mountain Dews, half the licorice, and about two to two and a half bowls of ice cream then fall into a sugar coma. I'm sure it's hard to believe but I had terrible acne, poor focus, and I was sick a lot. As a young athlete, I was also always dealing with sports injuries, probably because I was not giving my body the right raw materials to function properly.

My Turning Point

On my 16th birthday, I decided to quit drinking soda, started working out with weights and because I wanted to gain lean muscle I started to read about nutrition and supplements. I started to read all about exercise, nutrition, and supplements. My skin cleared up, my focus improved, I was sick less, and it was like a dark cloud was lifted. I don't care if you want to look better, feel better or perform better; you must start with your nutrition and whole food nutritional supplements. As much as I love to exercise, good nutrition is what has dramatically changed my life.

Look at Food Differently

Don't think of food as good or bad. Think of the hormonal response to eating food, meaning how your body responds to eating something. It is ultimately about chemistry, not calories!

Does your body respond favorably or unfavorably? Do you get tired, gassy, bloated, have joint pain or even a headache?

Ask this question to yourself; are you feeling better or worse than you did before you ate that food? You are either moving closer to or further away from your health goals by the hormonal response you have to your food.

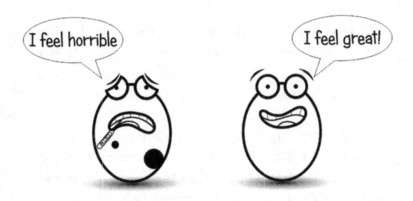

Food can either be like medicine
or like poison to your cells

Sherry's Success Story

Sherry came to us because she was having diarrhea every single day. She always felt like she was eating a healthy diet, but knew there must be something she was doing wrong.

After assessing her through MFT testing, we discovered that she had an intolerance to eggs and as soon as she eliminated eggs from her diet her diarrhea disappeared the next day.

I also have a story as it relates to eggs. Remember every body's biochemistry is unique to them. I was trying to gain some lean body weight, and so I increased my protein substantially. I was eating between 12 and 18 eggs every single day. Eventually, I would also develop an intolerance to eggs and to this day I still have problems if I eat eggs.

In fact one morning my wife had made me eggs for breakfast and shortly after I finished the meal I bent over and when I bent over my back hurt immediately. What had happened is the eggs created internal inflammation, and that internal inflammation caused my deep abdominal muscles to literally stop working, and I developed back pain that quickly.

Food can stay in your system up to 72 hours, so if you're eating the wrong type of food for your chemistry, you can have many different symptoms.

You could experience skin issues, digestive challenges, problems with your sleep, joint pain, clouded thinking and even migraine headaches; these are all symptoms that are many times directly linked to what we're eating. Your skin is the ultimate guide to tell the world how you are tending your garden. Know a kid with acne? Get them off sugar, wheat, and dairy and Voila!

Fix their gut, and you'll fix their skin.

Putting the Right Fuel in Your Body

If you had a high-performance sports car you would probably put high-performance gas in it, wouldn't you? If you put diesel in a vehicle that runs on gas, your car will malfunction and the longer the diesel sits, the more damage it can do to the fuel system, engine and injectors. I have no idea what that all means because I know nothing about cars, but that's what my brother-in-law Tim said would happen. But it sure doesn't sound great, does it?

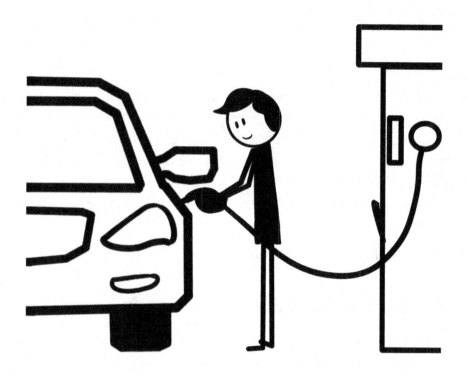

If you want to perform at a high level and look and feel a certain way, you have to put the right fuel in your body.

With so many different diets out there it can be quite confusing and frustrating to know what to do. Just because a nutrition program worked for your neighbor, co-worker, your favorite celebrity or your spouse, doesn't mean it's going to be the best plan for you. People are still hanging on and listening to outdated information.

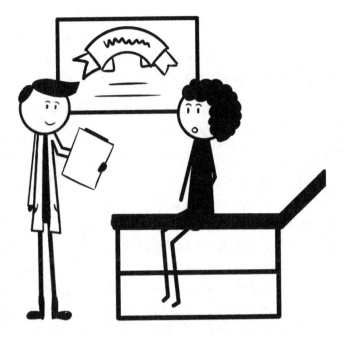

THE HIGH-CARB DIET I PUT YOU ON 20 YEARS AGO GAVE YOU
DIABETES, HIGH BLOOD PRESSURE AND HEART DISEASE, OOPS.

If I were to write the shortest nutrition book in history it would contain the following info;

Eight Simple Nutrition Tips

1. If the food wasn't around 500 years ago don't eat it
2. If it comes in a box, bag or wrapper don't eat it
3. If it's nonorganic don't eat it
4. Do eat lots of organic veggies, limited fruit
5. Do eat lots of good healthy fats
7. Drink half your body weight in clean, purified water with a pinch of sea salt added to it
8. Use whole food supplements to fill in your nutrition gaps

Keep this in mind; there is the factor of biochemical individuality. This means based on your genetics and other variables like the health and function of all your organs and glands, we all have individual needs.

Look at how different the diets of different cultures can be; compare the Inuit of Alaska with tribesman of Africa or South America.

The Inuit live off more protein and high fat versus more plant life and very little fat with various tribes in warmer climates. Our internal chemistry can be very different from others, with some people being more sensitive to certain foods. This is why at our wellness center we test our wellness clients to ensure they are putting the right fuel in their body. Doesn't it make sense to give your body the fuel that's right for you?

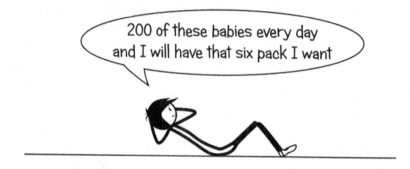

Is it possible to spot reduce? Ya know to crank out 200 crunches every night and flatten your stomach. What about doing 200 leg lifts to slim your thighs and butt or get rid of your flabby arms by doing lots of arm work. People still think they can spot reduce through exercise and I can tell you without hesitation, it's not going to happen! You have muscle, and you have fat. You can have beautifully developed muscles, but if you have a layer or two of fat over that area, nobody is going to see it.

All Calories are not Created Equal

A calorie is a calorie is a calorie is what I heard when I first studied nutrition in college. Originally I was taught the law of thermodynamics, and the basics are, if you want to lose one pound of fat in a week, you need to create a calorie deficit of 3500 calories because that's how many calories are in one pound of fat. So you determine how many calories you need to maintain your weight and then either burn 500 calories a day through exercise, restrict your consumption of calories by 500 or do a combo of both. Burn 250 and restrict 250 calories daily.

Let's do the math, 500 calories a day times 7 days in a week that totals 3500 calories and bam, 1lb of fat lost. Well not exactly. Why? Because hormones control what happens with our bodies. Remember earlier when we talked about the response your body has from the food you eat. Let's say you have a twin sister and you and your twin sister determine you need 2300 calories to maintain your current weight using that formula.

You both exercise and burn 500 calories a day on average, but what you eat daily is very different.

Your sister eats a bowl of whole grain cereal, toast, and juice, she then has a foo foo coffee drink later with a scone at a local coffee shop, pizza for lunch with coworkers and then because she has to run her daughter to dance and her son to baseball she stops and gets some fast food which consists of a cheeseburger, fries and a soda.

You start your day with a veggie omelet and a green juice, you bring a chicken salad for lunch, and you drizzle on some olive oil for flavor, you go home that night, and your husband is grilling the fish he caught yesterday, and you add a yam and some asparagus to the meal. Both of your daily calorie consumption adds up to 2300 calories. What happens over the weeks if you both eat similarly to this day and your calories expended are identical? Your body will respond very differently based on what you are eating. Chemistry kicks math's butt here!

Are We Psychic?

My wife and I can tell pretty quickly how a person's organs and glands are functioning, as well as, their sleep habits and even how they are dealing with their emotional stress. How in the world do we do that? Where you store your body fat is determined by two things, your genetics, and your body's hormones. Your hormonal response as it relates to how you exercise, what you eat, what time you sleep along with all your other stressors and lifestyle factors.

We have worked with hundreds of clients to actually help them spot reduce their trouble areas with specific nutrition and supplementation, but also, more importantly, help them restore optimal function to their specific organs or glands that were unbalanced. We call it Scientific Spot Reduction. As we improve the function of a particular gland or organ the stubborn body fat around that area magically disappears.

Hmm, where should I put this fat?

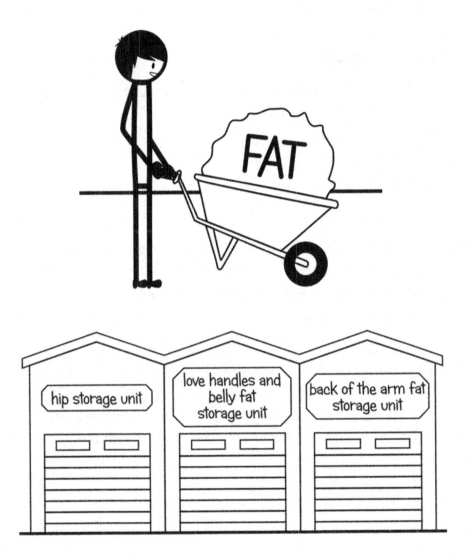

What your body fat storage says about you and your hormones.

Belly Fat Storage

Excessive fat in your belly region is an indicator of too much cortisol. What does cortisol do?

Cortisol is often called the "stress hormone" because of its connection to the stress response. However, cortisol is much more than just a hormone released during stress.

What Is cortisol?

Cortisol is one of the steroid hormones and is made in the adrenal glands (commonly referred to as your stress handling glands and they sit right above your kidneys).

What Cortisol Does?

Cortisol can help control blood sugar levels, regulate your metabolism, help reduce inflammation and assist with memory. It has a controlling effect on salt and water balance and helps control blood pressure. All of these functions make cortisol a crucial hormone to protect overall health and well-being.

Why I had to Fire a Client Story

Carrie came to see me specifically because she wanted to lose her belly fat. Carrie was a referral from a current client, but she lived over an hour away so we would be putting together a plan that she would follow on her own. When I asked her what she was currently doing for exercise, she told me she was exercising between two and two and half hours daily at her local gym. As she sat there in our appointment, she was fidgeting like a little kid, and she really lacked focus when I was asking her about her nutrition and lifestyle questions. After gathering all the information, I put a program together for her.

The first thing I did was cut her exercise time down considerably. I recommended breathing and foundational exercises that would cultivate energy for her, not deplete it. She was a total stress basket, and she was stressing her body more with all of her inappropriate exercises. I could see she wasn't thrilled with me cutting back her exercise even after I explained why she was storing her belly fat in her midsection.

My wife and I gave Carrie her plan and told her we would see her in a couple of weeks. When she came back, she said she wasn't noticing that much of a difference. I asked her to go over her program that we gave her so we could troubleshoot any problems.

She admitted she wasn't exactly eating what we had recommended and she didn't always remember to take her supplements. Carrie also admitted she had added some extra cardio classes to what I recommended. I asked her why she did that. She just felt that she needed more exercise to get better results. I told her what she was doing was no longer our program, and she had already proven her formula didn't work.

I explained again her body needed to cultivate energy and not deplete it anymore. Her stubborn body fat was not going to leave her body because it was acting as a buffer to protect her from all the toxins in her body and her type-A plus personality was cranking out too much cortisol.

I gave her some tough love and sent her on her way and told her I would see her in a couple of weeks again. She came back, and it was pretty much the same story. I told her we could not be responsible for or attach our name to someone's health and fitness results that are not going to follow our program. My wife and I take our reputation for producing positive results very seriously, and we are not afraid to fire a client.

One of the hardest things as caring practitioners we had to learn was to never be more invested than the client. Everybody must take responsibility for their health and fitness, but everyone needs good coaching to guide them along the way. My wife and I receive coaching every year ourselves by experts that know more than us in their respected fields, so ultimately we help more people get better and quicker results.

Love Handles and Upper Back Fat

If you store your body fat here, then you have insulin or sugar handling problems. This pretty much means you don't handle carbohydrates well.

Hips and Leg Fat

If the back of your thighs have a lot of fat, it indicates a high level of exposure to environmental estrogens and a poor ability to detoxify them once they are inside the body. Women are exposed to much more toxicity on a daily basis than men because of things like toxic personal care products.

High body fat on the front of thighs indicates that your body is producing too much estrogen.

Back of Your Arms

Women and triceps fat are closely linked to liver toxicity. This doesn't mean your liver is failing, but you have accumulated enough toxins to start affecting your hormonal and metabolic functions.

Men and a high percentage of triceps fat are linked to how much testosterone a male has.

Fat Storage at the Side of the Rib Cage

This indicates how well your thyroid is functioning.

A blood test will not always give an accurate picture of the functioning of your thyroid because a blood test is more of an end-stage test. Body fat storage and MFT testing are much more accurate.

We have clients that say they had their thyroid tested via a blood panel and it was fine, only to be experiencing symptoms galore of a poorly functioning thyroid.

When we have a client that is unbalanced hormonally, food alone will generally not do the trick to restore their balance. This is when we need to have a very specific custom supplement program for them. We have all heard the saying, "you can't always judge a book by its cover", but in regards to where someone stores their body fat as well as looking closely at a person's face using Chinese face mapping we can tell a lot about their health. We then get very precise through our assessments.

I'm going to say it again, "If you're not assessing you're guessing and do you really want to guess with your health." If you are going to spend any time, money or energy on improving your health why not get a custom plan?

So can you spot reduce troubled areas? Yes and no. Not by exercise, but you certainly can with the right nutrition and supplementation program. Find someone you trust, get some sort of evaluation as to what your nutrition and supplement needs are and then follow the program. Unless you would rather just guess what your needs are. If that's the case, good luck with that!

We, of course, use MFT as our testing method; you could also do other forms of muscle testing, saliva, stool and urine testing, and even hair tissue mineral analysis through a holistic health practitioner.

Repeat after me, "If I'm not assessing I'm guessing and my health is way too important to me to guess, I want to get to the root cause and create optimal balance in my body. How I look, feel and perform with my body comes down to balance in and with my body."

So take care of your garden, quit with the math and learn about your chemistry!

Chapter Four

Supplements

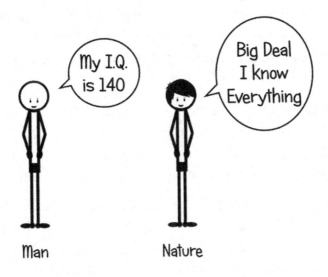

Who is Smarter Man or Nature?

Man will never outsmart nature. Manmade supplements are inferior to whole food supplements, and generally, you should always be taking whole food supplements. There are applications for synthetic supplements, but why are you guessing with your health. Get tested regularly to ensure you are on the right program. Otherwise, you are just potentially wasting money because there are way too many variables that go into what food and supplements you currently need.

Think back to all the stressors; food, heavy metals, chemicals, scars, structural and emotions. Your stress load determines your need for your nutrition and supplements and the raw materials (nutrition) you feed your cells are the most important factor in your health.

It could be argued that never in history has so much money been spent on the advertising and purchasing of any merchandise, with so little knowledge of the product itself, on the part of either the seller or the buyer, as has been spent on vitamin and mineral supplements.

Most people don't know how supplements are made, their characteristics, their attributes, their sources, their uses, their advantages, and disadvantages, and how to tell one from another by reading a label.

Two of the top selling supplements in the United States are; One a Day, a product family of multivitamins produced by the Bayer corporation. The second one is owned by the pharmaceutical giant Pfizer, and it is Centrum. Imagine that, the top two vitamin supplements are owned by drug companies. The average person will absorb about 3-5% of that garbage, and the average consumer has no clue about this.

With rare exception, these types of supplements draw energy away from your body rather than providing energy to your body. Almost always the energy signatures of these supplements are mismatches to the M-Field.

What is the Difference Between A Natural and Synthetic Supplement?

In short, it's the difference between something that's living and something that's dead.

That's a big difference!

NATURAL WHOLE FOOD VITAMINS

On vitamin labels, the word "natural" has no specific definition other than that the substance exists somewhere on the planet or in outer space.

The key words to look for are **"Whole Food Vitamins"** – this means vitamins as they are found in food, untampered-with in any way that would change their natural structure, their biological or biochemical combination, or their actions.

> Vitamins in their natural state always exist as living complexes with specific nutrients to really work, like enzymes, phytonutrients, and organic minerals, and never as isolated single factors. **A vitamin needs all of its "family" to function.**

Organic food sources are preferred since they are most nutrient-dense and contain no pesticide residues.

CRYSTALLINE means that a natural food has been treated with various chemicals, solvents, heat, and distillations to reduce it down to one specific "pure" crystalline vitamin. In this process, all the synergists, which are termed "impurities," are destroyed. There is no longer anything natural in the action of crystalline "vitamins" – they should more accurately be termed drugs.

SYNTHETIC means that a chemist attempted to reconstruct the exact structure of the crystalline molecule by chemically combining molecules from other sources. These sources are not living foods, but dead chemicals. For example, Vitamin B1 is made from a coal tar derivative, and d-alpha tocopherol (so-called Vitamin E) is a byproduct of materials used by companies to make film. However, it is not legally necessary to give the source from which the synthetic "vitamin" is derived. Synthetic "vitamins" should more accurately be called drugs.

HOW TO READ A LABEL To identify synthetics on the label, look to see if a source is given. If it isn't, assume the product is synthetic. These terms also identify a vitamin as synthetic:

- Acetate
- Bitartrate
- Chloride
- Gluconate
- Hydrochloride
- Nitrate
- Succinate

Whole-food natural supplements never come in high dosages. It is only possible to create high-dosage "vitamins" if you isolate one fraction of the vitamin complex like they do in synthetics.

THE FALLACY OF "HIGH DOSAGE EQUALS HIGH PO-TENCY" Consumers have been thoroughly fooled and misled about vitamins. We have been brainwashed into believing that large quantities of dead chemicals are more nutritionally potent than smaller amounts of high-quality living compounds.

Relatively small amounts of whole food natural vitamins, with all of their naturally occurring helpers, are far more potent than high doses of synthetic imitation "vitamins." (Think of it this way. If you were in a fight would you want to go it alone or have your whole family backing you) Synthetic=isolation and Whole Food=integration of all the "family of nutrients" otherwise known as synergists.)

Do Synthetic Vitamins Function As Well As Natural Whole-Food Vitamins?

Living systems are even more complex and specific in their need for building materials. Also, living systems are constantly breaking down cells, organs, and tissues, and rebuilding and repairing them. For these processes, the body must have a continual supply of high-quality material.

The body has a very precise design which is so incredibly intricate and complex that even with all the scientific and medical research thus far; we have only scratched the surface of understanding it.

What arrogance it is to think that man can alter a design we don't even understand.

Many conventional and even alternative healthcare practitioners think that there is no difference between natural and synthetic vitamins, or between naturally chelated minerals and inorganic minerals. This is incorrect and has led to enormous confusion in the nutritional field.

The following examples are a handful of nuggets that I found to make this point:

- Reported on April 14, 1994, in The New England Journal of Medicine was a study in which 29,000 male smokers were given synthetic beta-carotene and synthetic Vitamin E to evaluate the cancer-protective effect of the "vitamins". After 10 years, the men taking the synthetic beta-carotene had an 18% higher rate of lung cancer, more heart attacks, and an 8% higher overall death rate. Those taking synthetic Vitamin E had more strokes.

Food source of these same nutrients, such as fruits and vegetables, consistently demonstrate protection against cancer, heart disease, and stroke.

- On November 23, 1995, the following was reported in The New England Journal of Medicine: 22,748 pregnant women were given synthetic Vitamin A. After four years the study was halted because of a 240% increase in birth defects in babies of women taking 10,000 IU daily, and a 400% increase in birth defects in babies of women taking 20,000 IU a day.

Women eating natural food sources of Vitamin A showed no increase in birth defects.

- Reported in Reuters Health, March 3, 2000, was a study of men who took 500 mg of synthetic Vitamin C daily. It was found that over an 18-month period, these men had a 250% increase in the inner lining of the carotid artery. This thickening is an accurate measurement for the progression of atherosclerosis. This is, synthetic Vitamin C induced atherosclerosis, even at a 500 mg dose.

Whole-food Vitamin C protects and repairs the inner lining of blood vessels, and is preventative against atherosclerosis.

Cookie Cutter vs. Customization

IN SUMMARY

You can't repair and rebuild a living body with dead chemicals, it simply isn't possible. As I stated earlier, even though we recommend and use whole food supplements almost exclusively, we will sometimes use a synthetic Pharmaceutical Grade vitamin and or supplement, but it must be more than 99% pure. This means there are no binders, fillers, dyes, or unknown substances.

However, most people read an article about some supplement or take advice from a friend or family member and then just take it; with no regards to if it is even something their body really needs or is their current priority. You can guess with your body or assess what your needs are based on how you are currently feeling or performing. Think cookie cutter vs. custom. What makes more sense to you?

Our wellness clients that are really committed to long-term health and function get tested every two to four weeks. Why would we recommend this? Because your stressors are always changing, meaning your nutritional needs are always changing! Most people just take a shotgun approach. Don't leave your health to chance, find someone who can test you on a regular basis and make sure you are giving your body the right raw materials to feed your precious cells. Remember, you can be proactive or reactive with your health.

As important as whole food nutritional supplements are in your diet because **everyone** is deficient in something, you still need to lead with good organic food. Sometimes when we put our clients on their custom supplement protocol, they will ask if they can take less than we recommend. One look at their nutrition log and the quick and easy answer is no! Why? Because the worse your food quality is, the more stress is put on your body, which in turn increases the need for key nutrients. You can't just eat crappy and then expect to make up for it with your supplements.

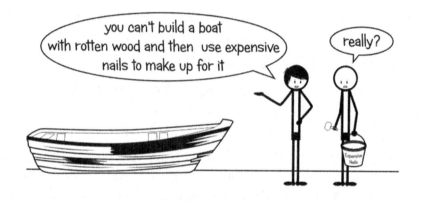

Eating crappy food is like using rotted wood for building a boat and then trying to make up for it by using golden nails. Not gonna happen!

Always lead with high-quality organic food and use whole food nutritional supplements to help rebalance your body.

Chapter Five

Dr. Quiet and Optimal Breathing; the Drug of Choice

My doctor has me on Ambien to sleep,
Adderall to focus, Ritalin for energy
and Xanex to relax and 8 other
drugs just for the side effects!

Why don't you just learn to
breathe properly,
no side effects
and the same results!

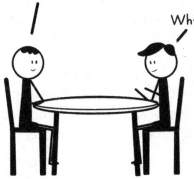

The World Health Organization has stated that by 2020 worldwide depression and anxiety will be the number one disability. In the United States, twenty-five percent of women are now taking anti-depressant medication, and anti-anxiety medication and men are close behind.

The CDC has also declared that sleep dysfunction is now at an epidemic level.

Imagine for a moment there was a drug that had no side effects and it gave you more energy, improved your mood, helped you sleep, made your eyes brighter, improved the look of your skin, strengthened your immune system, improved your focus, and helped eliminate joint pain and headaches?

Well, that drug doesn't exist, but you can still get all those benefits from just learning how to breathe properly again. The reason I say again is because when you were a baby you just naturally breathed correctly. Unfortunately, through poor posture, stress, and injury, you start to pick up bad habits that can really affect your health negatively.

Poor breathing mechanics can lead to depression and anxiety, low energy and major sleep issues. Joint problems like neck, jaw, shoulder, lower back pain, headaches and even numbness and tingling in the hands often have their roots in poor breathing mechanics.

If I could teach only one subject in regards to health and fitness, I would definitely choose breathing. Most people are very surprised by that because people don't think that there's really anything they can do to change their breathing.

Over the years I have never evaluated a client who could not significantly improve their breathing from a health and fitness standpoint.

Breathing is both a conscious and unconscious activity, and throughout the course of the day most people aren't paying attention to how they breathe, but you can control how you breathe, and it can have a very dramatic impact on your health and fitness.

There are so many different types of breathing and also so many different applications to optimize both your health and fitness. You can slow your respiration down to control stress, and you can also energize yourself and increase mental clarity in just a couple of minutes with various breathing techniques.

You can also breathe at a specific tempo for enhancing sleep at night. There are so many incredible benefits to breathing properly. Yes, breathing has a tremendous amount of benefits, but done incorrectly breathing can lead to a whole bunch of joint problems.

Did you know that 90 percent of the population is breathing at just about 50 percent capacity? By the age of 50, we lose about 40 percent of our breathing capacity, and 92 percent of the world has poor air quality. Poor breathing mechanics literally cost this country billions of dollars because of all the negative things it can be attached to.

The Fairy Tale that Almost Never Happened

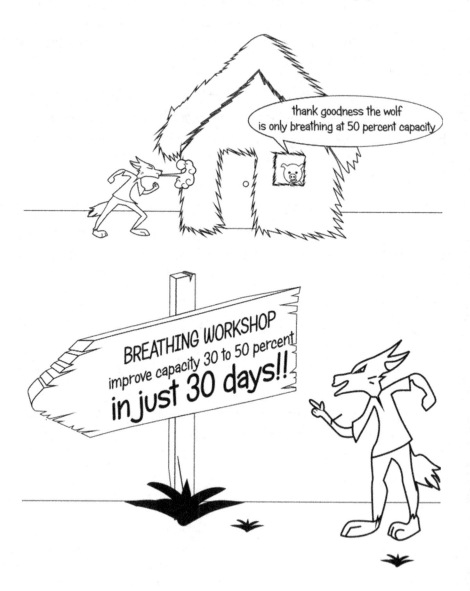

30 days later...

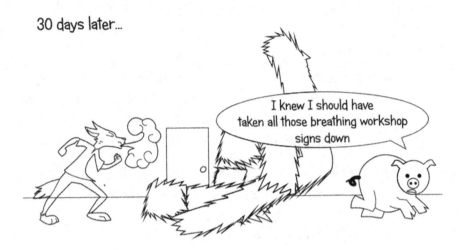

There are so many strikes against the average person when it comes to breathing, but you can see amazing and dramatic results in just 30 days. Just ask the wolf!

Based on my clinical experience I believe that breathing is one of the most critical, fundamental and foundational things that you can do to optimize your health and fitness.

As a Holistic Therapist and certified breathing coach, one of the first things my team and I evaluate is how someone is breathing. I think breathing should really be the foundation of all therapy and fitness programs because it is such an integral part of how human beings should move and very rarely is it ever talked about.

The average person breathes approximately 20-25,000 times a day. When you breathe that many times, you either have an opportunity to enhance your health or you have an opportunity to actually create some physical problems.

Try this experiment; fold your arms how you typically fold your arms, now try and switch the position of your arms the other way.

For most people, that feels very foreign and the reason it feels very foreign is because you've established a specific pattern. What happens when you establish these patterns are your nervous system, and your muscles adapt to these patterns.

It can take as many as 5,000 repetitions to learn or unlearn specific patterns, so if you are moving incorrectly (like breathing), you have to be consciously aware of how you're moving. Then you need to learn to fix your faulty mechanics.

If you need to hire a breathing or movement specialist, it's worth the investment if you have any dysfunction that is creating pain or other symptoms.

Are You Breathing Correctly?

I want to invite you to take three big breaths. Go ahead and take three deep breaths and really pay attention to what's going on in your body. C'mon set the book down and do it.

When the average person breathes one of the things they notice is they get taller, and they lift their rib cage up. Those people can be referred to vertical breathers.

When you become a vertical breather, you can really overwork your accessory respiratory muscles. These are the muscles that elevate your shoulders, and when they are overworked, it can lead to upper body joint pain, like jaw, neck, and shoulder as well as headaches.

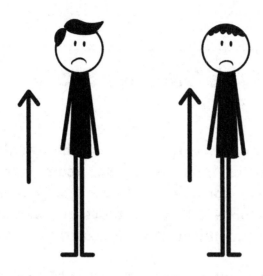

ARE YOU A VERTICAL BREATHER

When you are a vertical breather, you're not originating your breath from your diaphragm which is your primary respiratory muscle.

There are many people who suffer needlessly with a lifetime of orthopedic problems because they aren't breathing optimally. I see people every month that have been to several doctors and therapists for the same joint pain because they have just been isolating the pain in their upper body.

If you don't fix your faulty breathing mechanics, you will just always be chasing the pain. I think it's very important that you learn how to reestablish good sound breathing mechanics or find someone that can coach you on how to breathe properly again.

Lisa's Success Story

Lisa had been having pain around her shoulder blade for a little over two years, and it was pretty constant. Lisa was going to her chiropractor two to three times per week for relief for 6 months just so she could function.

When I evaluated Lisa, I noticed right away she was a vertical breather. I explained to Lisa she had just been chasing her pain and until she corrected her breathing, she would continue to do so. As I shared with her the other muscle imbalances she had and why she had them and how we would correct them she had a rush of emotions.

Lisa was excited that the information made so much sense, and she believed our staff could help her get rid of her awful pain, but she also became very upset that the other three practitioners she saw for this were just doing things that made her feel better temporarily but didn't correct her problem.

I understood what she was feeling because I had also spent a lot of time, money and energy trying to fix some of my issues over the years, but you can't go back, and you hopefully learn from it.

Within 5 sessions Lisa was pain-free, and after 10 sessions she made major posture changes, and she restored her breathing mechanics to optimal. She also said her stress level went down considerably and her ability to deal with certain situations with her young children was like night and day. As she said, she had more bandwidth to cope.

Ultimately you want to initiate your breathing from your diaphragm, fill your lower lungs and then finish filling your upper lungs. When you learn to become a horizontal breather, your whole health and fitness picture changes for the better.

But there's something more interesting that I have found teaching people how to breathe. There's a tremendous relationship between breathing and emotions. I want to tell you a story about your lungs and grief.

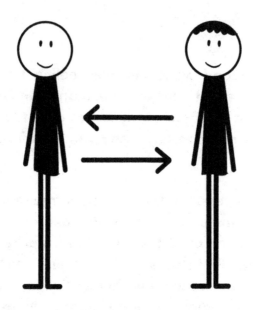

ARE YOU A HORIZONTAL BREATHER

Tom's Success Story

This happened when I gave a talk to about 50 people about happiness, breathing, and anxiety. After the talk, I left the building and went down to my car. The CEO followed me out, and he said look I'm 58 years old and I started having panic attacks for the first time in my life.

When you're a CEO having panic attacks doesn't work, you can't sit in a board meeting and suddenly feel your neck get stiff and a splitting headache coming on, and you want to run screaming out of the room.

What should I do? I asked him when did these panic attacks start? Six months ago. What happened six months ago? He said my brother died. And you were close I said. Yes very. And you're a workaholic aren't you? And he smiled and said yes. After the funeral, you went right back to work.

And he said yes. I said you don't have an anxiety issue, you don't have a panic attack issue, you have a grief issue. You haven't grieved the death of your brother. When you suppress grief, which you've learned to do, and you keep suppressing it, it begins to layer as new events begin to happen in your life and it comes out in another way, it comes out in anxiety.

Your panic attacks are happening because of your grief. So what should I do? Work with me for a few sessions, and I'll show you some breathing exercises that will help correct this.

Today Tom has no panic attacks, they've stopped completely, and he is feeling great.

Tom realized that he really didn't grieve his brother, so by allowing himself to feel the grief which most people are terrified of, his anxiety is gone!

How Do I Release Emotion from the Past?

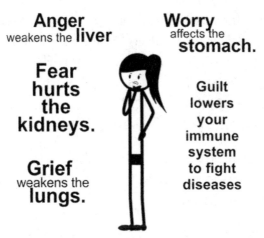

Anger
weakens the **liver**

Worry
affects the
stomach.

**Fear
hurts
the
kidneys.**

**Guilt
lowers
your
immune
system
to fight
diseases**

Grief
weakens the
lungs.

Why do so many of us suppress grief? Because we're taught that expressing grief is socially unacceptable, but most people will express anger much more readily than grief.

We will shout at the TV screen if our team is losing, we'll even yell at another car and not apologize to the passengers in our car. But if you start crying when you're talking to someone, you wipe your tears away quickly and say, I'm sorry I don't know where that came from.

Of course, men are bigger culprits than women because we've been taught that's it's a sign of weakness and failure. If we were very honest with ourselves, we wouldn't teach our children to live the way we are. We wouldn't say, go to the best school, get a great job and then live on sleep medication, anti-anxiety drugs or pain killers.

It's not what we want to teach our children, but through our actions, that is what we're teaching them. It's quite interesting.

If you're under stress, if you want to sleep better, if you want to become energized and if you want to improve your health and fitness you have to make a conscious effort on focusing on how you're breathing. There are specific techniques in how you can optimize the functionality of all those things I mentioned just by learning how to breathe properly!

You can go from a fight and flight state (sympathetic or breakdown) to rest and digest (para-sympathetic or rebuilding state) in about ten breaths.

When life gives you lemons, just take a few deep diaphragmatic breaths and then go make some lemonade.

Chapter Six

Joint Pain and Posture

Today in spite of the fact that we have more clinics, doctors, therapists, and technology than ever before millions of people suffer needlessly in pain. People come into our wellness center every week and say the same thing, "I've tried everything, and I still have pain"; they're tired of it, and for some, they have determined it must be old age or genetics or just the cards they've been dealt. They've checked numerous boxes on their list of things tried: ice, heat, bracing, rest, therapy, cortisone shots and even surgery.

Upon closer review most of them haven't tried everything; they have just done the same three or four things over and over and expected a different result. They've tried a LOT of things, but haven't tried it all. They've done multiple therapy techniques, and some of them even had multiple surgeries. They've bought high-end chairs, purchased a standing desk as well as cut out various forms of exercise they believed to be causing their pain.

Yet, they haven't done something as "simple" as returning their body back to its original design.

Posture and Pain

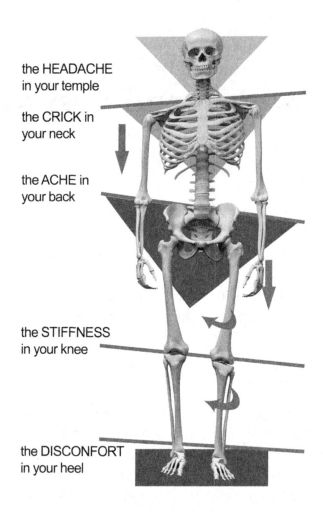

the HEADACHE
in your temple

the CRICK in
your neck

the ACHE in
your back

the STIFFNESS
in your knee

the DISCONFORT
in your heel

Fix Your Frame
Fix Your Pain!

When you are in pain, your body is doing something it's designed to do, so you try to pay attention and hopefully correct your underlying problem. Your job is to find smart people who understand the real CAUSES of muscle/joint pain and give you the solution.

I am always amazed when I ask clients what types of exercise and stretches they did for their therapy and then what they tell me. Based on what I hear from clients there are generally two major things that are wrong with the therapy programs they went through.

The first thing is their injury or dysfunction is isolated or compartmentalized by only focusing on their structure and not all the other stressors that are playing a role in the pain or dysfunction. Rarely is a joint problem ever a single variable and because conventional physical therapy only addresses the structural piece, many people will just not get better.

Not enough therapists know how to assess postural imbalances (or length/tension relationships) that ultimately lead to joint pain. When I have clients demonstrate some of the exercises they did in therapy they will often demonstrate something like a level four exercise. Later when I evaluate them, they can't even do a level one exercise correctly. So not only are the exercises in my opinion misprescribed, but the client cannot even execute the exercise with good sound mechanics and sometimes these people have worked with three or four therapists.

I think to get the best results people need to really understand why they are in pain or what caused their dysfunction. I have found over the years the more a person understands their imbalance, the more compliant they are and ultimately the better results they achieve. Rarely do doctors or therapists really do a good job of explaining why their client/patient is in pain and what they are going help them do to fix the problem.

Some of the things clients tell me are things like, "I felt overwhelmed because the therapist gave me four or five exercises in a 30-minute session." "They just gave me these handouts with pictures of the exercises and showed me how to do them, but they didn't spend that much time showing me how to do them, so I wasn't sure if I was doing them right." "I did exactly what they told me to do and didn't get any better."

Years ago posture and muscle imbalances were at the forefront of orthopedic examinations, but now a person is sent for x-rays, an MRI or CT Scan and a quick consult with an orthopedic doctor. When it comes to any level of joint pain, the first thing I look at is a client's muscle balance or posture to determine if the muscles surrounding the joint are doing their job.

Your muscles not only move you around but also act as shock absorbers that are designed to absorb force. It doesn't matter if that force is a bag of laundry, a child, lawn furniture, a jet ski or even your own body weight, force is a force. If your muscles aren't handling that force where's it going?

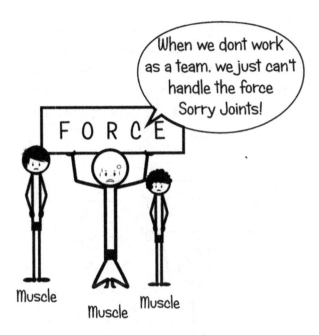

Think of the muscles that surround any of your joints as three people rowing a boat. What happens when one guy stops rowing? The other two have to row that much harder. What about if two people stop rowing? The third guy becomes overworked and can no longer handle the stress or the force.

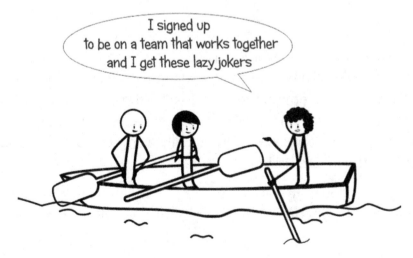

When the muscles that surround a joint don't work together as a team or unit, that particular joint does not function properly. That joint will also take on the stress the muscles were supposed to take on. That stress is going to be absorbed by soft tissue such as tendons, ligaments, fascia, nerves, synovial membranes and even discs. So what happens next? That's right, your joints are stressed.

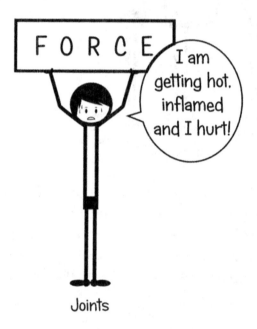

Joints

What does the average person do when they have an inflamed joint? They take an anti-inflammatory which long term can lead to problems in their gut. Maybe they get a massage or ice, brace, stretch and even just rest. The question is, "Are the getting to the root cause and actually fixing the problem that created the inflammation?"

Now if you remember the cool chart that my wife and I created? FYI Chapter 2 is where it's at for review. Remember all the variables that can stress out your nervous system and lead to inflammation? Foods, Immune Challenges, Chemicals, Heavy Metals, Emotional Stress, and Scars. Very rarely is it just a structural issue, this is why so many people bounce from doctor to doctor and therapist to therapist and never really get "fixed"

Conventional medicine isolates the symptom and looks at the problem as a part, instead of looking at your whole system.

Think of a skeleton, better yet, think of your skeleton. Your skeletal frame work is moved by your muscles which are getting the command from your brain through your nervous system. So your joints or your skeletal frame work is controlled by your muscles and your nervous system.

Your Nervous System, aka "Big Daddy"

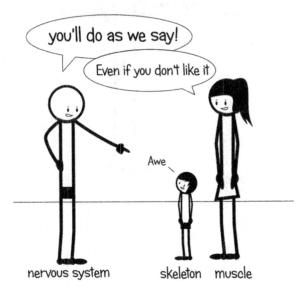

Your skeleton is under the control
of your nervous system and muscles

So if there is something that's stressing out your nervous system and your muscles aren't working the way they're supposed to, then the stress will end up in whatever joint that is moved or stabilized by those muscles. That could be your shoulder, your back or your knees. Why? Because your muscles aren't doing their job of absorbing the force or stress, so it ends up in your joints.

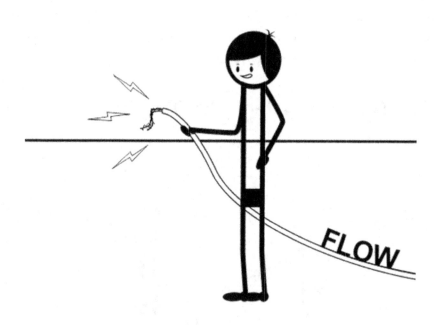

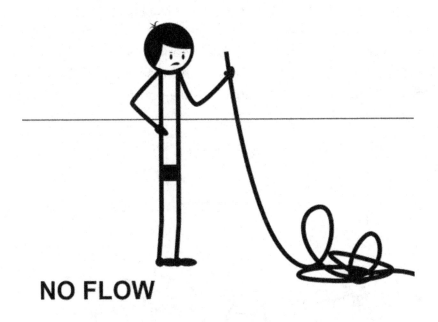

NO FLOW

Let's think of your nervous system like a big electrical cable. When you have flow, your muscles and organs will work properly because the nerve "feeds" them, so to speak. When you don't have flow through your body as you remember, bad things happen. If you don't have flow, are your muscles or organs going to get stronger or weaker? Yes, you are exactly right if you said weaker.

Symptoms, dysfunction, and disease all have their roots in limited or no flow, an imbalance in your body and poor cellular communication. Remember that your nervous system is the "Big Daddy" and when your nervous system is stressed your muscles are not going to work the way they are supposed to and that means joint stress and potential joint pain.

Muscles, Organs, and your Nervous System

Let me give you an example with low back pain; now stay with me on this one. If you raise your arm out to the side, you are able to do that because your brain sends the message via two different nerve signals, a primary and a secondary. So it's like your shoulder has two brains, but are you ready for this, your abdominals have nine sources of nerves.

Your abs essentially have nine little brains.

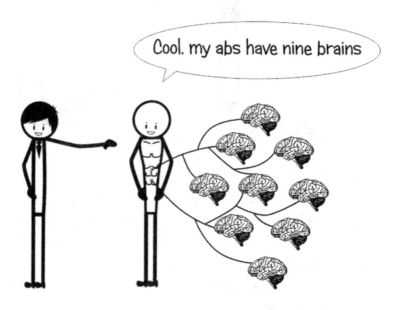

Now, why is it so important to know this? The reason so many people that suffer from low back pain never ever get better is because most conventional treatment programs only focus on the structure of the back and this is known as isolation. It's crucial the six other categories of stressors (foods, immune challenges, chemicals, heavy metals, emotions, and scars) that can irritate and stress out your nervous system are addressed, or they will shut off your abdominals' brains, weaken your muscles and create low back pain.

It doesn't matter if you have a food intolerance, irritable bowel, constipation, loose stool or inflammation coming from your sex organs, this inflammation will turn off the muscles that stabilize your back and pelvis. For men and women, scars are a biggie; a surgical scar, an episiotomy, cesarean or a hysterectomy scar can all stop nerve flow creating low back and hip pain. Not to mention something that plagues almost 50% of all women over 38 years of age, urinary incontinence.

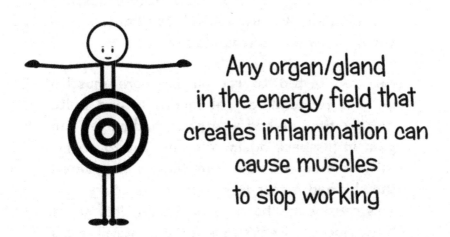

Any organ/gland
in the energy field that
creates inflammation can
cause muscles
to stop working

Kent's Success Story

Back pain, scars, and prostate.

Kent came to us because he had a history of chronic lower back pain and was really struggling when he came in. When we initially assessed him, we realized his deep abdominal stabilizers were not firing/working, and therefore his spine was unstable. He also had a lot of tightening in the muscles that surrounded his hip.

As we started to retrain his core muscles he was responding real favorably and quite quickly, then he had a setback, and he felt the pain in his back again. We had yet to do his MFT assessment; when we did, we discovered that he had a scar from a hernia surgery that was causing his hose to be kinked (his nerve flow blocked. Kent's muscles that stabilize his spine quit working again. We addressed his surgical scar with a cold laser and wheat germ oil, and that deactivated his scar and increased flow again to his muscles. Kent immediately

started to respond again, and his back pain disappeared.

Then once again he had a setback. When we tested him again using the MFT technique, my wife discovered he had a bacteria on his prostate. Anything within the energy field that creates inflammation can cause a muscle or organ to be stressed, and they don't work the way they are supposed to.

So once we addressed his surgical scar and the bacteria on his prostate, he immediately gained control of his major spine stabilizers, and his back pain was completely corrected. At the same time, we probably prevented something more serious with his prostate. This was a classic situation where he would have been chasing the pain of his back forever, never "fixing it" because conventional therapy methods would have only addressed the muscles and the joint.

After 12 years of chronic back pain and working with multiple doctors, drugs, and therapists, Kent finally got to the root cause of his problem and fixed it!

Muscles are married to the same organs that they share nerve flow with, so if a guy has inflammation with his prostate or a woman has inflammation in her ovary, there's going to be problems. If someone has a food intolerance, they're bloated or gassy, any other of these stressors it could cause the deep spine stabilizers to be shut down and not work properly. Just knowing this is a game changer. Hopefully, you will now first ask yourself, "Self, what do you think is stressing out my nervous system?"

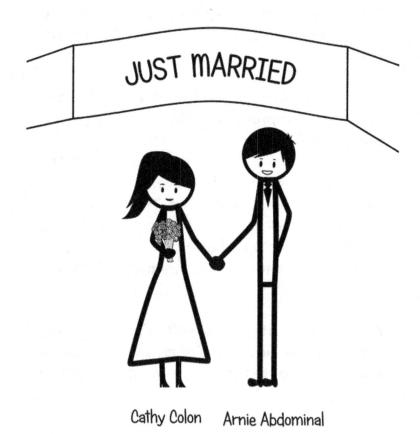

Cathy Colon   Arnie Abdominal

The Fairy Tale That Didn't Make the Cut but Should Have

I didn't think my daughter Sydney could benefit from the fairy tale Goldilocks and the Three Bears, so I changed it a little bit. Some of you are probably thinking this alone could have had me nominated for father of the year.

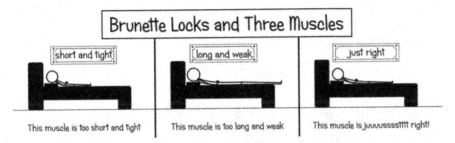

Brunette Locks and Three Muscles — short and tight | long and weak | just right

This muscle is too short and tight | This muscle is too long and weak | This muscle is juuuussssttttt right!

These are the three muscle patterns Brunette Locks found:

Certain muscles in your body under stress will become too short and tight, and other muscles will become too long and weak. When muscles get short and tight, those muscles called the Agonists shut down the muscles on the other side called the Antagonists and then they get long and weak.

Think short tight muscles on the front of your hips and thighs and wimpy, flabby butt! What's happens? Those muscles can no longer absorb force. So again, the stress is going to end up in your joints and with this example, pain in your back or hips.

When it comes to exercise most people focus on looks instead of building a great foundation, i.e... Optimal posture. Posture isn't just for looks; good posture will keep you pain-free and performing optimally which will allow you to move with ease and grace regardless of your age.

When you have balanced posture, your muscle lengths are juuuuuussssstttt right!

Surgery and Automobile Tires

Let's say your tires on your car are wearing unevenly, and you go to get some new ones. When you get there, the service person at the tire store checks your alignment, and they determine your alignment is way off. What do you do, just go ahead and only get the new tires?

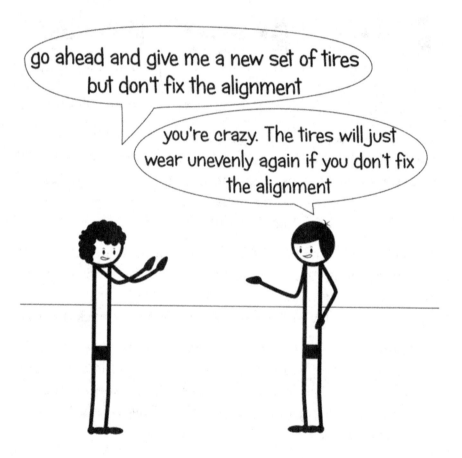

What happens with most orthopedic surgeries? Because the muscle imbalances were never addressed, the muscles that surround that joint are still not working the way they are supposed to, so the joint will just end up taking on the stress even after surgery. The stress will either end up in that same joint, or you will just end up compensating, and this ultimately leads to inflammation in another joint. My staff and I have saved literally hundreds of people from having to have surgery.

I have news for you if you go consult with a surgeon he/she is generally going to recommend surgery. You can take 100 people, 40 years old and over, off the street that are completely symptom free in regards to joint pain and you will find the following issues if they all had some type of imaging like an MRI, CT Scan or x-rays: Bulging discs, disc herniations, degenerating discs, cartilage fraying and arthritis. Let's say you're in pain and have imaging done. Now the doctor shows you conclusive evidence that you have an issue, they use a lot of big Latin words which you don't understand, and then they tell you why you have to have surgery.

The doctor has a fancy office, multiple degrees and they have shown you proof that you need surgery or else.

I know this story plays out because I have heard my clients tell it to me over and over. I tell them they have nothing to lose if they approach it holistically. If it doesn't work for you, you can comfortably tell yourself you really did try and then have the surgery. There certainly are times when orthopedic surgeries need to be performed, but in my opinion based on thousands of hours of clinical, in the trenches proof, it is very rare they need to be performed. When we restore our client's muscle imbalances many times, their pain completely vanishes, and their performance improves dramatically.

Imagine building your dream home. You have everything in the blue prints you ever wanted and then some. Inside you have marble floors, Persian rugs, the finest custom cabinets, high-end fixtures with smart technology that can control every function in the house with just the touch of a button. You cut no corners except when you built your dream home; you built it on a weak foundation. What happens? Disaster!

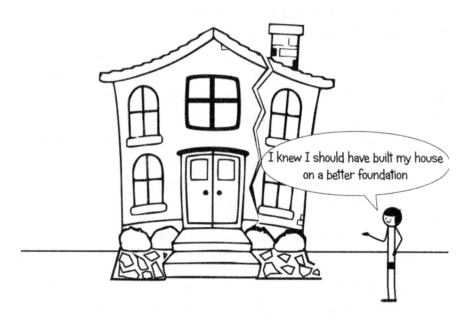

Most people are motivated by their outward appearance, and the first thing they want to address is their body fat and building and toning some showy muscles. They join a gym because they want flat abs and toned arms. They give no thought to their breathing or posture and very few trainers ever even address these things with clients. This is why to look better with exercise, so many people end up getting hurt.

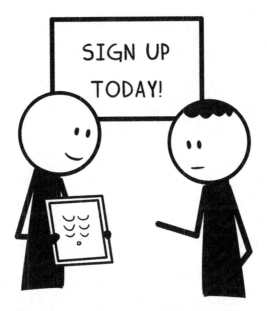

YES NIK, OUR QUICK START GYM MEMBERSHIP COMES WITH A FREE SET OF PRESS-ON ABS!

But the secret to a pain-free and high functioning body is to take the time to first plan how to build a solid foundation. You do this by learning how to breathe correctly, and then you address all your muscle imbalances, so you can look, feel and perform your very best. Restore function first, your body will thank you for it!

Chapter Seven

Dr. Movement and the Power of 7

Even though you now understand the importance of building your foundation we will be reviewing some of the key areas. We are adding different categories to ensure your exercise program has everything you need to perform at your highest level. Seven is the magic number when it comes to fitness.

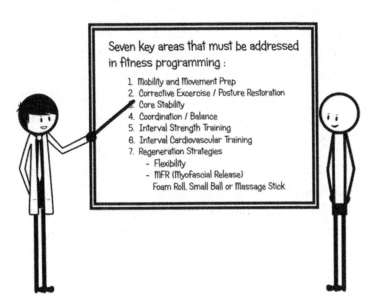

Seven key areas that must be addressed in fitness programming :

1. Mobility and Movement Prep
2. Corrective Excercise / Posture Restoration
3. Core Stability
4. Coordination / Balance
5. Interval Strength Training
6. Interval Cardiovascular Training
7. Regeneration Strategies
   - Flexibility
   - MFR (Myofascial Release)
     Foam Roll. Small Ball or Massage Stick

Number one: Mobility and movement prep

Of course, people are familiar with general flexibility information and simple stretches, but most people don't talk about mobility exercises. However, it is better to be slightly tight regarding your flexibility and have an optimal range of motion in your joints.

It's important that you articulate or move your joints through a full range of motion for each joint, or if the joint has been damaged approach the optimal range of motion every day for good joint health.

Have your joints ever just felt stiff? Why is that? As we age we develop scar tissue and calcium deposits within our joints. Joint mobility exercise stimulates and circulates the joint fluid, which 'washes' the joint. The joints have no direct blood supply and are nourished by this synovial fluid, which simultaneously removes waste products that are in the joint.

Joint salts or calcium deposits are dissolved with the same gentle, high-repetition movement patterns. Properly learned, joint mobility can restore complete freedom of motion to your ankles, knees, hips, spine, shoulders, neck, elbows, wrists and fingers. It's especially important to keep your spine mobile and free, and if there were such a thing as a fountain of youth, joint mobility exercises come very close.

As I have gotten older, joint mobility has become more and more important because of the damage I had to my joints from all the years of abuse playing sports. If I am ever pressed for time and have to shorten my workouts, I never shorten my mobility and warm up work because safety is the most important factor in my workout. You can't get more fit if you are hurt!

You can use mobility exercises as your warm up, an active recovery during other activities, or as a stand-alone workout. One of the things I do every day is to start my morning with joint mobility and breathing because it just gets me going and feeling like I'm ready to start the day.

No matter how tired I am, when I do energy breathing techniques along with joint mobility, I am ready to perform at a high level in minutes.

When it comes to exercising at the gym, people tend to get on a treadmill, an elliptical or a stepper if they're going to do any type of strength training as part of their warm up. It's important that you warm up your body in all three planes of motion to prepare yourself for the exercise that you'll be doing.

You should always mobilize your joints and take them through proper planes and ranges of motion before you do any type of exercise. So, for instance, you can do shoulder circles, arm circles or hip circles, squats, and side and forward bends. The important thing is you try and move each one of your joints through a full or optimal range of motion each day for at least a few repetitions.

Integrating joint mobility exercises into my fitness completely changed how my body functions and it has dramatically decreased my pain along with improving my performance. If you don't know how to perform joint mobility exercises, find someone that can show you how to perform them correctly.

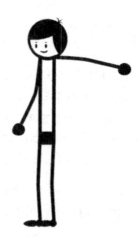

Mobility is the oil for your "Inner Tin Man"

I personally don't go a day without mobilizing my joints, and it is how I and all of our clients warm up before our workouts.

A general rule of thumb when it comes to joint mobility for joint health is to move each joint through its optimal range of motion as many times as you are of age. So if you are 50 years old, move that joint 50 times through the optimal range, or if that joint has been damaged, try and approach optimal range and then increase the rep range to 100-200 repetitions. This will lubricate the joint and break up scar tissue as well.

Number Two: Postural restoration or corrective exercise

Of course, we covered this in the last chapter, but I really want it to sink in. Typically when people go to the gym, they exercise muscles that they can see. For instance bicep curls or a front raise, this is where you raise your arm to the front of your body, but most people need at least a 3 to 1 ratio of training their backside to their front side. For most people to restore balance back to their bodies, they need to do more exercise with the muscles that they can't see. If you are working with a trainer or therapists that is something that should always be incorporated into your routine.

Number Three: Core stability

As you know it is important to support and stabilize your spine, remember your spine is not designed to be load bearing. Your spine is merely an anchor point for the muscles and the ligaments. Studies have demonstrated with as little as two and a half pounds of pressure your spine can be damaged, so if your deep core muscles are not functioning the way they're supposed to, it's very easy to hurt your back.

So what is the definition of the core? The definition of the core is really everything minus your arms and legs. It is incorporated in almost every movement of the human body.

Many of the muscles are hidden beneath the exterior musculature people typically train. The deeper muscles include the transverse abdominals, multifidus, diaphragm, pelvic floor, and many other deeper muscles. All human movement starts from the core. It is critical to your health and fitness that you ensure you have fully functioning core muscles. As a point of reference, of the thousands of people I have evaluated, I had NEVER tested someone that had a fully functional core when they started with me and that includes Olympic and professional athletes. But fear not, you can restore your core; you just need to start with your foundation and then build out.

What the Core Does

Your core most often acts as a stabilizer and transfers force, rather than just move your body. Yet consistently people focus on training their core in isolation. This would be things like doing crunches or back extensions versus functional movements like deadlifts, overhead presses, squats, and pushups, among many other functional exercises. When you exclusively exercise on machines not only are you missing out on a major function of your core, but also better strength gains, more efficient movement, and longevity of health.

I have tested hundreds of people with a flat stomach, or even six pack abs and they still have low back pain. Why? Because the small stabilizing muscles underneath the big mover muscles are not working to stabilize their spine. Very rarely are they breathing properly which adds to their dysfunction.

Professional Dancer Success Story

One of our current client's daughters is a professional dancer in New York. Shelly was having low back problems and was going to be in town for a few weeks performing, so her mom asked if we could assess Shelly's back. She had already worked with the production team doctor, another orthopedic doctor along with seeing three other physical therapists and still no relief. Shelly had a beautifully sculpted dancer body with washboard abs.

When I was taking her through her assessment, I felt there was something around her belly button. I asked her, "Is this a belly button ring?" Sure enough, it was. When we tested Shelly using MFT, we determined that her belly button ring was stressing her nervous system out and shutting down her deep core muscles and that was creating instability in her spine leading to painful movements.

Shelly removed her belly button ring, then we spent a couple of sessions re-educating her deep abdominal muscles so they would work the way they were supposed to. Because Shelly had compensated for so long, when we first started, the most basic moves were tough for her and humbling. As a high-performance dancer with very good body awareness once it all connected with her she responded quite quickly. Back pain was gone. Simple fix if you know what to do.

Shelly then asked me, "I live in New York, the biggest city in this country and these doctors and therapists had all the credentials, so why couldn't they help me?" What I told Shelly is, If you don't live in the Holistic world of therapy, a lot of people are just going to fall through the cracks because many times they are only dealing with the structural component instead of looking at all the variables that stress out the nervous system.

Number Four: Coordination and balance

Most people neglect any type of coordination and balance. People tend to gravitate towards things like walking on a treadmill or on an elliptical machine and strength train on machines, so they never really challenge their coordination and balance systems. Most of the strength training we do at our wellness center is done standing rather than seated which is a big difference from sitting on a machine.

Footwear is so important regarding coordination, balance, and stability when you're exercising. You have small little sensory organs in your feet that tell your brain where you are in space and the thicker the sole of your shoes the more it will retard the messaging to your brain. Running shoes are for running, not for strength, balance and coordination training. The flatter the shoe's sole the better when you are doing any type of strength training as well as balance type exercises. Training barefoot is also a great way to train coordination and balance.

Number Five: Strength Training/Metabolic Resistance Training (MRT)

You can go to any gym in the world, and you will find very, very few people that exercise with good sound exercise mechanics. We always tell our clients it's vitally important they perform their exercise with great mechanics, and they should be aesthetically pleasing to the eye when they exercise. If you're executing an exercise and you don't look good doing it, it's probably not going to feel that good at best, and at worse, you are going to get hurt eventually!

For instance, if you really round your back when you lift an object off the floor, you increase the likelihood of really hurting your back. If you don't understand proper lifting mechanics, it's important that you meet with someone to show you how to exercise safely and correctly. When you exercise properly, you are not only safer but also more efficient, and that should be your goal.

Ask yourself this question when working out? "Am I getting the most value for my investment of time and energy?" Most people that work out are just going through the motions and don't really understand the technique and how the exercise should feel. You should always feel like you are in control of the exercise rather than having the exercise feel like it's controlling you.

Mastery vs. Variety

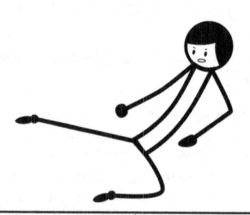

I fear not the man who has practiced 10.000 kicks once.
but I fear the man who has practiced one kick 10.000 times
– Bruce Lee

I remember having a conversation with one of our trainers, Nik, about people mastering good exercise technique, "Most people are more interested in variety than mastery." These people will never be efficient in their workouts, and they will always be more vulnerable to injury. I think one of the things I am the proudest of is looking around our fitness studio and watching our clients that exercise with us executing beautiful form with their exercises.

We are fortunate to attract clients with great focus and desire to be as safe as possible while getting the most out of each exercise. They probably have better exercise mechanics than 99% of the general exercise population because we work so hard at it. I go to different gyms all the time to do, shall we say "research" and I am always amazed at the horrible form I see and this includes people working with trainers.

I especially love when our clients travel and go to an exercise class in another town and then come back and tell us, "You guys would not believe how bad the form of some people was and the trainer didn't even fix it." Our clients are developing critical eyes for good form, and that gives me a big warm and fuzzy feeling!

If you are truly focused on mastery, it's impossible to get bored, and the probability of injury lowers significantly. I have been strength training for over 30 years, and I am still in search of the perfect rep myself because I am always trying to make my workouts more efficient and safer.

What is Metabolic Resistance Training (MRT)?

MRT differs from your standard weight-training session, but the results are far superior in how it can improve your fitness. It's an intense form of resistance training that engages your whole body through a full range of basic well-designed movements such as squatting, deadlifting, lunging, pulling, pushing and twisting. Essentially you are going from strength exercise to strength exercise in a circuit fashion with no/limited rest between exercises.

How to Burn Fat Longer with EPOC and MRT

EPOC stands for Excess Post Exercise Oxygen Consumption. This means your metabolism is elevated for as long as 30 plus hours after your workout, now I like the sound of that don't you?

MRT is a time-tested way to burn fat faster — it's much better than jogging and other forms of more conventional "cardio. It's a demanding workout style, but well worth the effort and you'll build yourself some functional, head-to-toe strength and fitness at the same time.

The good thing is, this method of exercise can be done in as little as 30-40 minutes, and you will still get incredible results if you're ready to put the effort in.........that's a promise.

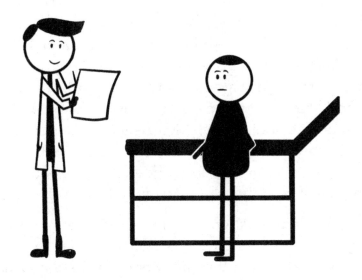

WHAT FITS YOUR BUSY SCHEDULE BETTER,
EXERCISING ONE HOUR A DAY OR BEING
DEAD 24 HOURS A DAY?

Number Six: Interval Cardio Training

Cardiorespiratory exercise is a term that best describes the health and function of the heart, lungs and circulatory system. The goal of any cardio workout should be to get as many large muscles working as possible. They not only need to work hard, but continuously, to burn the greatest amount of calories during and after exercise.

How much is too much? The Concept of "Smart Cardio":

It is important to perform "smart cardio" because your body quickly adapts to cardio-based workouts. The more you do, the more efficient your body becomes, causing you to burn fewer calories from your fat stores each time you exercise.

Because your body adapts so quickly, cardio-junkies are forced to adjust their workouts to last increasingly longer to provide the same calorie burn. This not only increases the amount of time you have to spend in the gym but also increases the odds that your body may start breaking down muscle instead of fat for fuel. Additionally, the benefits are temporary. Aerobic activity doesn't increase the amount of fat you burn after your workout like resistance training does. Your metabolism returns to normal shortly after stepping off the treadmill.

Smart Cardio will greatly enhance the rate at which your body burns calories. The most effective Cardio programs are designed around the **HIIT Principle. I am constantly in search of producing the best results with the least amount of work.**

One of the buzzwords in fitness and weight loss circles is High-Intensity Interval Training or HIIT. This method of exercise has the potential to allow an exerciser to lose body fat faster than any other form of "aerobic" exercise, because of EPOC.

Although interval training is not a new concept in the field of sports conditioning, it has become a popular exercise style for general conditioning and weight loss. Just to give you a visual on the benefits of intervals think of the Olympic track sprinters. They are very lean and muscular because this is how they train. Now think of the Olympic marathoners. Some of them look like they are haven't eaten for weeks. In my opinion, they look weak and frail. Compare them to the sprinters who look, healthy, strong and vibrant. Sprinters do short and intense intervals, and the marathoners do long slow distance work.

What is HIIT?

Intervals involve performing bouts of high-intensity work (20 seconds to as much as 3 minutes) separated by recovery periods of about 2-3 times the duration of the bout. Since most casual exercisers may never have done intervals, it may be helpful to use a perceived effort scale of 1-10 to regulate intensity; with 1 representing little effort, and 10 representing absolute maximal effort. Aim for about 8-9 on the effort scale.

So if you are using an exercise bike: after warming up for about 8-10 minutes, do a burst of 30 seconds as hard as you can. Then rest for 2-3 minutes and then repeat for 5-7 intervals. Then, cool down at a low intensity for about 5-10 minutes (This is just one example of how to do intervals)

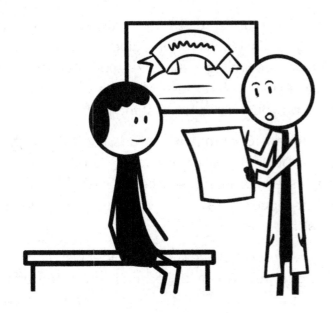

I RAN A DISTANCE OF 15 BLOCKS TODAY.
THEY WERE LEGO BLOCKS, BUT IT'S A START!

HIIT spares muscle and maintains metabolism

Intervals help avoid the muscle wasting effects associated with continuous low-intensity exercises such as jogging and walking. Intervals help spare valuable lean muscle mass which is a key determinant of your Resting Metabolic Rate. Simply put, lean muscle gained will cause you to expend more energy even while you sleep!

Number Seven: Regeneration strategies

My favorite techniques for flexibility are:

SMFR (Self Myofascial Release)

AIS (Active Isolated Stretching)

To understand myofascial release, we must first understand fascia. In keeping this "science lite," imagine a very strong dew-covered spider web encircling a shrub. And between the gaps in the threads is a clear gel, rather than air. If you can picture this, then you're on your way to understanding fascia.

This three-dimensional matrix threads itself throughout your body, surrounding your muscles, organs, nerves, bones, blood vessels and even our cells. Everything is held together and in place by fascia. It is impressively flexible and infinitely adaptable.

Fascia is a very strong, very connected spider web and when one spot on it gets tugged or pulled or injured, the effects ripple throughout the body. This is why you may have pain in your knee that may have nothing to do with a knee injury, but everything to do with an injury to your lower back. The natural, fluid state of the fascia has been traumatized, causing it to harden and tighten.

Ever pull a thread on a sweater only to find the whole thing bunching up on one side? That bunching is exactly what happens to fascia when your body experience stresses, whether it's dehydration, injury, inflammation, repetitive activity—you name it.

Your body reacts to pain of any kind by creating a protection response, that while, initially is a good thing, over time can lead to increased pain, build up of toxins and reduced blood flow and oxygen to the area. When you experience a slight amount of tissue damage—this can be due to a physical injury, or a psychological one like depression, or even something like an ulcer—pain signals are sent to the spinal cord which then triggers the muscles around the injury to contract in order to provide support and protection for the surrounding tissues.

This response, left unchecked, creates a vicious cycle of pain as more blood flow is restricted to the contracted area. More signals are sent, and more muscles tighten to protect the growing area of pain. What may have started as something small has now grown—that sweater gets more gnarled and bunchy.

Myofascial release (MFR) is designed to go in and smooth out those hard knots, returning your fascia to its normal fluid and adaptable self.

But how?

MFR, a gentle, sustained pressure is applied to points of restriction (those bunched up tender spots), allowing the connective tissue to release. Picture a stick of cold butter. If you jab your finger into it sharply, you're just going to hurt your finger, and not even make a dent in the butter. But if you place your finger on the butter, and apply gentle pressure, you'll find you're able to slowly sink into the stick of butter, melting your way into it.

This is essentially what is happening when you perform Self Myofascial Release (SMFR) with tools such as foam rollers and massage sticks and balls. Self-massage is one of the best things you can do pro-actively for the health of your muscles and joints. I never travel without my massage stick and massage balls.

Flexibility...

It's one of the most coveted attributes of human movement whether you are young or old, but the traditional methods for attaining it fall short for most people.

You probably remember your high school gym teacher making you sit on the floor of the basketball court, open your legs, and then try to get your head as close to the floor as possible. But no amount of effort ever seemed to get you any closer, so you moved on and resigned yourself to being stiff.

Or maybe you kept working at it for years as part of a sport or fitness class. And maybe you even made progress, but it wasn't easy. In any event, you've probably decided that stretching doesn't work very well for you. If you cannot attain a position you'd like, then you need to find a way to get to that range of motion.

A Quicker Solution for Better Flexibility

Active Isolated Stretching (AIS) is a technique that helps people maximize the effectiveness of stretching without causing the sort of discomfort that keeps a lot of us away from it.

AIS is a specific technique that uses four basic principles:

Isolate the muscle to be stretched.

Repeat the stretch eight to 10 times.

Hold each stretch for no more than two seconds.

Exhale on the stretch; inhale on the release.

Seems easy enough, right? Let's look at some of the details that make AIS so effective.

How do we isolate a muscle to be stretched? Isolate the muscle to be stretched by actively contracting the opposite muscle. Let's say you want to stretch your hamstrings, (the muscles on the back of the thigh) you must first actively contract the quadriceps (the muscles on the front of the thigh). Then, the brain sends a signal to the hamstrings to relax. This provides a perfect environment for the hamstrings to stretch.

What is the purpose of repeating each stretch? Repeat each stretch 8 to 10 times to increase the circulation of blood, oxygen, and nutrients to the muscles being stretched. This technique will help you gain the most flexibility per session. Remember, the more nutrition a muscle can obtain and the more toxins a muscle can release, the faster the muscle can recover.

Hold for two seconds. How does that help? Each stretch is held for a maximum of two seconds to avoid the activation of the stretch reflex. The stretch reflex prevents a muscle or tendon from overstretching too far or too fast. This reflex is like putting the parking breaks on your flexibility. This is our body's natural protection against strains, sprains, and tears. By holding short-term stretches, we increase our range of motion with each repetition and eliminate any fear of pain, and we take the parking brake off.

Breathing is an essential component to decrease fatigue in the muscles. Muscles need oxygen to function well. If there is not enough oxygen, lactic acid is created. Lactic acid creates that sore feeling in our muscles. If our muscles are sore, they are less powerful, more fatigued, and more prone to injury.

After a long hike, walk, or strength training session what are the problems that pop up and keep you from going out again? For most of us, it's the same patterns: sore muscles, old injuries, and new injuries. These things make it hard to go out and have fun while training.

Active Isolated Stretching can help your training and recovery become more efficient and more fun, and it is far superior to holding a static stretch for long periods of time. If you are looking to quickly and safely increase your flexibility make sure you incorporate SMFR and AIS. Who knows with a little work we may just see you in Cirque du Soleil.

Seven Movements You Must Have in Your Fitness Programming

These foundational exercises must be included in your strength training routine. It's important that everyone squats, bends, pushes, pulls, twists, lunges along with walking, jogging or sprinting. The reason why those foundational exercises are so important is that is precisely how the human body is designed to function. If you take a look at people that live in third world countries they move their bowel from a full squat, they work from a full squat, they cook from a full squat, and they hang out in a full squat because they don't have chairs. They sit on their haunches.

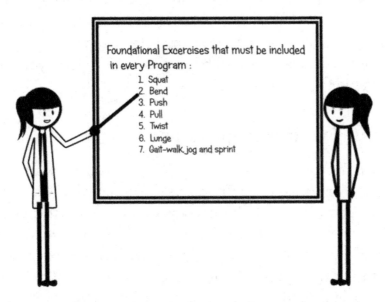

Your body is designed to be able to do a full squat. The reason why most people can't is that they quit doing it. Most people sit a lot and then that increases the tightness in their hip muscles and they lose the ability to do a full squat. The squat is the most important of all the movements because of all the benefits it provides.

The big difference between functional movements and machines is you're not working in three-dimensional planes with machines. You don't have to coordinate or balance when you're on a machine, so those systems within your body become retarded because they're not stimulated.

Your body is not designed to work in isolation; it is intended to operate in integration or as a team. Your muscles should work together to move your body and stabilize your joints to keep you safe from injury. The more you isolate your muscles like a bodybuilder, like on a machine then, the more dysfunction that you can develop. If you train only on machines your global muscles or your primary mover muscles become stronger in relationship to your small stabilizing muscles leaving you more vulnerable to injuries and joint pain.

Is Your Exercise Appropriate For You

Many times people will ask me what do you think of some particular exercise or method. It's important that we qualify this question. You really have to ask yourself, not is this a good or bad exercise or method, but is this appropriate for me and my current abilities. So not only do you have to execute the movement with good mechanics so you can be efficient, but it's also important you pick appropriate exercises for your own safety.

One of the reasons why I have such good exercise form and why I am more efficient than 99% of the people that workout is I am not afraid or embarrassed to do a push up on my knees if that's what it takes. I will regress back to the next easier version of any exercise if I have to, so eventually I will get the most out of that exercise.

When I go to other fitness facilities, I see people literally making up exercises, or they're following routines or exercises that they have no business doing just because they saw it in a magazine or they saw someone else do it. There are also many times I see other trainers using inappropriate exercises with their clients. It's leading to a lot of injuries today because people are not staying within exercises that they have the ability to perform safely. Make sure your workouts are about you and your level and don't compare yourself to others. There are too many variables to judge yourself against others, so don't do it!

Does Your Doctor Know Squat About Exercise

Many times people will come into our wellness center, and when we start talking about exercise, they say, "yeah I really like your philosophy when it comes to exercise, but my doctor said I shouldn't squat."

So the question I have for them is, "well then how do you move your bowel, how do you sit in your chair, how do you get in your car?" I'll then ask them to demonstrate their squat. When they do most of the time, their form doesn't look pretty, and I can clearly see that they have quite a few muscle imbalances that are causing them to squat incorrectly. Remember when your muscles aren't doing their job of absorbing force, that force is going to go into what? That's right, your joints! See how much you know now.

What I usually say is, "what your doctor should have said is, "you shouldn't squat like that." I have never found anyone in 23 years that I couldn't get into a full squat if they were committed to doing so. I've had people that have had hip replacements and knee replacements, as well as back surgeries, get in a full squat with their thighs below parallel.

As long as they were committed to working on it, we just slowly progress them down into a beautiful and functional squat. If you go to third world countries, you'll find people in their 80s and 90s that can do a full rock bottom squat where they're literally sitting on their haunches.

Remember to always exercise at your level and always pay attention to the details so you can have a safe and efficient workout.

Chapter Eight

Science Helping Nature to Heal and Balance Your Body

The world is held together by electromagnetic fields. Your body is electromagnetic and every function is an electrical event, which starts in your brain and travels through your nervous system. You actually have over 45 miles of nerves in your body, in fact, if you took everything away from your body except for your nervous system, you would be able to make out the form of your body because of how vast your nervous system is.

Batteries, Cells and Your PH

Your body is like a battery, and your cells have a measurable electrical charge which gives you the ability to repair an injury and fight off disease. When your cells are adequately charged your cells can perform tasks like injury repair much quicker and with higher levels of effectiveness. In the nutrition chapter, we discussed chemistry over mathematics, but true health is really about electronics and energy which is physics.

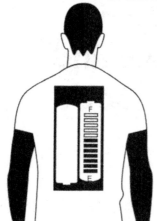

All life is energy
... and all energy is electromagnetic.

- The cells in the body require electricity.
- When the cells drop their electrical charge to a certain level, they comeback sick.
- The first sign of illness is usually pain.
- Chronic Disease & Pain is always defined by low electrical charge.
- The body can heal almost anything with proper nutrients and electrical charge.

How does your cells' energy become low?

1. Mineral levels get low due to nutritional deficiencies
2. AC/alternating current (found with alarm clocks, laptops, cell phones, power lines and TV's) is electronic pollution to your body and is everywhere draining your body's DC or direct current.

We've all heard the saying you can either be part of the problem or part of the solution. Well, there are things in your life that either move you closer to or further away from optimal health. In my nutritional microscopy training we learned that all disease occurs when you are acidic; what this is really saying is that all disease occurs when your voltage is low, or you're in what can be called an electronic stealer state.

Low Voltage=Pain and Sickness at the Cellular Level

Electron Stealer (Think muggers stealing someone's purse or bad guys)

- Causes damage
- PH 0- 6.9 (PH stands for Potential Hydrogen)
- Acidic
- Has a positive charge
- Is Destructive
- Has low voltage

In my training, I even heard the statement, alkalize or die. Translation, you must have electrons available to do work, or your cells will die. Excuse me while I take a sip of my green drink which is very alkalizing and is an electron donor and has high voltage.

High Voltage=Pain Free, Healthy, and Vibrant at the Cellular Level

Electron donor (Think someone giving to someone in need or good guys)

- Can do work
- PH 7.1–14 (Optimal health is about a PH of 7.3)
- Alkaline
- Anti-oxidant and has a negative charge
- Constructive
- Has high voltage

How Do Your Cells Normally Get Voltage?

Because of the fact, the earth is a giant electromagnet; if you take a volt meter and stick the electrodes into the dirt, you would be able to measure voltage. With today's toxic environment, it is a big challenge for the health of your cells. Electrons (otherwise known as voltage) will always flow from an area of high voltage to an area of low voltage. So, if your body has a lower voltage than the earth (think massive charging station) walking barefoot on the dirt or grass will cause electrons to flow from the earth into your body. It's literally like plugging you into your very own cellular charging station.

This connection is referred to as Earthing or Grounding. By walking **barefoot (shoes will not allow for this)** on grass, sand, dirt or rock, you can really diminish chronic pain, fatigue and other ailments that plague so many people today. Your connection to nature, the planet, and the universe is so important to your health. However, with advances in technology and our modern, fast-paced lifestyles, many of us have become separated from our basic bond with Mother Earth.

We all know that the sun gives us warmth, light and vitamin D and the Earth provides us with fresh air, water, food, and a surface to live on. But not many people know when your bare feet make contact with the Earth's surface your body uptakes a natural and subtle energy which could be referred to as vitamin G – G for ground.

Throughout history humans walked, sat and slept on the ground, cultivated their land with bare hands and spent a lot of their time naturally grounded. Unfortunately, we have become increasingly disconnected from nature by our modern lifestyle.

Conductive leather-soled shoes of our ancestors have been replaced with insulated rubber and plastics. We sleep in beds and homes off the ground. Plastics, synthetic fabrics, asphalt, tar, carpets, vinyl have all been introduced and block this natural connection. We are also bathed in electron stealers like household appliances, mobile phones, wi-fi, microwaves and cell towers. These things bombard us continuously with excess damaging charges which affect both our tissues and cells.

The Earth's energy helps to knock these excess damaging charges down so that your body can heal and repair naturally, as it is meant to. Therefore, to remain in good health, it is imperative that we reconnect with this natural energy daily to counteract the damaging effects of our modern lifestyle. While typing this book, I have repeatedly taken breaks and went outside in my bare feet and stood in the grass and just breathed from my belly and yes it did feel great, and it was a total recharge!

Skip the Pretty Shoes and Go Barefoot

Go barefoot outside for at least a half-hour and see what a difference it makes on your pain or stress level. You can sit, stand, lay or walk on grass, sand, dirt, or plain concrete. These are all conductive surfaces from which your body can draw the Earth's energy. Wood, carpet, asphalt, sealed or painted concrete and vinyl won't work and will block the flow of electrons as they are not conductive surfaces. Experience for yourself the healing energy of the Earth at work next time you are stressed, in pain or not feeling well.

I just got back from a hike out on a trail that I have hiked hundreds of times and came across a woman who was hiking barefoot on the trail, and I had to talk to her. I have seen thousands of people on this trail over the years, and while I am writing this chapter I meet a woman barefoot on a trail, you can't even make this up. Usually, when I go hiking I am in a zone, and I move pretty fast, but I had to find out why she was barefoot.

She had been walking and running barefoot for the last year and told me she can't believe how much better she feels since she started going barefoot. She has less joint pain, more energy and she said she definitely feels calmer. She used to suffer from anxiety and doesn't anymore. (Little did she know she was going to run into Larry King on the trail?) I couldn't believe how excited she was to share her experience of earthing and she had an incredible energy with calmness at the same time. Very cool.

Free electrons (think recharging your battery) are taken up into your body, and these electrons could be referred to as nature's biggest antioxidants that help neutralize bad stuff in your body that can lead to inflammation and disease. This could be the difference between you feeling good or not so good, having a little or a lot of energy, sleeping well or not so well or looking vibrant or looking tired and old.

Your body is composed mostly of water and minerals which in combination are excellent conductors of energy from the Earth, provided there is direct skin contact for them to flow through. When your cells have a healthy electrical charge, your body has the energy to cope with mental stress and the ability to repair your cells. No matter what your age, gender, race or health status you will benefit from a daily dose of Earthing!

Some Benefits Earthing Has Been Shown to Help With:

- Help with the cause of inflammation, as well as improve or eliminate the symptoms of many inflammation related disorders
- Reduce chronic pain
- Improve Sleep and promote a deeper sleep
- Increase energy and vitality
- Lower stress and promote calmness in your body by cooling down your nervous system and stress hormones.
- Thin your blood and improve blood pressure and flow
- Relieve muscle tension and headaches
- Lessen hormonal and menstrual symptoms
- Dramatically speeds healing time
- Reduce or eliminate jet lag
- Protect the body against potentially health disturbing electromagnetic fields (EMFs) such as computers, alarm clocks, cell phones, etc.
- Accelerate recovery from intense athletic activity

Not only is the Earth like a giant battery charger, so are all living things on the planet, including us as individuals. A lot of our clients at our wellness center will tell you I give out and receive a lot of hugs. I come from a family of huggers, you know the people that stand at the door and hug each other for 30 minutes saying goodbye.

Remember that voltage moves from an area of higher voltage to an area of lower voltage, so when you hug someone, the one with the lower voltage will get a donation of electrons from the other one and if you would continue to hug you would soon be at the same voltage. I can imagine you thinking the next time someone is hugging you that you will feel all tingly inside knowing they just donated an electron or maybe you did, even better! This process works the same way with any living thing that you touch; for example, if you hold a dog or cat and you're at a lower voltage than the dog or cat will donate electrons to you, then they will run outside recharge itself and bring some more voltage to you. If you lean against a tree, the tree will donate voltage to you, even moving water will because it is always an electron donor. Still, water is an electron stealer, taking a shower will energize you while a bath will make you tired. Swimming in the ocean will give you electrons, but swimming in a chlorinated pool will steal voltage from you.

Common ways electrons are stolen from your body:

- Acid water (think tap water)
- Carbonated beverages, alcoholic beverages
- Cooked food
- Processed food
- Root Canals
- Mercury Fillings
- Moving air: the wind, air-conditioning, fans, convertibles, and hair dryers

It is all about the cells

What does a cell need to stay healthy?

1. **PEMF** - Significantly increases the cells electrical charge & magnetic energy, allowing it to repair & regenerate.

2. **H2O** - Drink half your body weight in ounces.

3. **Good Quality Macro Nutrients** - Carbohydrates (sugars), Lipids (fats), Proteins.

4. **Micro Nutrients** (vitamins & minerals) - Organic, Non GMO, Natural Supplementation & Good Quality Salt.

5. **Oxygen** - Excercise / Movement This increases your O2 levels.

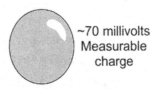

~70 millivolts
Measurable
charge

Healthy Cell

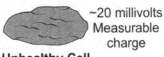

~20 millivolts
Measurable
charge

Unhealthy Cell

Sometimes Our Bodies Just Need A Little Help

Energy always flows between all your cells. When damage or trauma occurs to living tissue, there is a disruption in the electrical capacity of the involved cells. After an initial surge, there is a measurable decrease in the production and flow of energy through the electrical network of the involved tissues. This condition is generally followed by pain in the area and often results in the body's inability to completely repair itself. Remember flow = health and no flow = pain and sickness.

Jake's Success Story

Jake was a 16-year-old baseball pitcher who was a referral from a current client. Jake's mom was worried and heartbroken for her son about the news they had just received and was telling one of our clients about the news. Jake had seen two orthopedic doctors about his painful elbow, and the last doctor said that he was born with an extra muscle in his forearm and it was creating his severe nerve pain. Jake couldn't throw a baseball without pain, he couldn't do any pushups, he could barely even open a doorknob because the pain was so bad.

Jake was facing a serious surgery and at least 4-6 months of rehabilitation with no guarantees of complete recovery and full function. He would miss all of his upcoming season plus have to deal with all the challenges that come with a major surgery. Our client urged Jake's mom to have her bring Jake in so I could evaluate him. After the assessment that I took him through, I found that he had a tremendous amount of scar

tissue surrounding the area creating pain and dysfunction.

So we supported Jake nutritionally to decrease his inflammation, and then our staff and I worked on him using microcurrent. Within about five sessions he was completely pain-free, and we went on to do five more sessions to completely eliminate any scar tissue that was around the area. So not only do we get him out of pain but we got him to a very high level physically.

Had Jake undergone surgery he still would have had the underlying dysfunction that created the pain in the first place.

When a cell is injured, diseased, or toxic, electricity and blood flow goes around the damaged tissue instead of through it. This is when the technological advances of specific frequencies and specialized equipment known as Frequency Specific Micro Current can dramatically accelerate healing of unhealthy tissue.

The electrical currents in microcurrent instruments seek the abnormalities of diseased, injured, or toxic tissue in your body and opens up the cell, enhancing nutrient intake and the elimination of waste products. The advanced microcurrent instruments that we use in our wellness center are input as well as output devices.

With this technology, the equipment can find the abnormalities caused by injury, disease, or toxins and then send out a corrective signal until the injured or unhealthy area is normalized electrically. Now blood can flow into the injured, diseased, or toxic area instead of going around it. This enhances the body's ability to heal itself in an accelerated manner, as cells reach a state of homeostasis, with no discomfort, side effects, overdoses, or over-stimulation.

Many kinds of therapy treat the symptom—most often pain—rather than the problem. Frequency specific microcurrent therapy goes directly to the cellular level where illness and injury begin.

Our bodies function through low-voltage conductivity. Currents flow through connective tissues, including muscles, tendons, ligaments, bone, and nerve pathways to the brain. When a person or animal is injured, its body's normal conductivity becomes altered.

Microcurrent therapy can speed the healing process and provide pain relief by improving the cellular metabolism of injured tissues. This is accomplished by applying a specific frequency of tiny electrical impulses to the cells of an injured nerve, joint, muscle, or tendon using simple probes via contact with the skin's surface.

Other forms of electrical stimulation treatment, such as with TENS (Transcutaneous Electrical Nerve Stimulation) devices, differ from microcurrent therapy. The electrical stimulation produced through TENS devices does not therapeutically treat the injured area. Rather, the device sends an electrical stimulation that blocks the sensation of pain from being sent to the brain.

Frequency specific microcurrent (FSM) devices are designed to read your body's response to electrical stimulation at the cellular level and adjust the electrical current sent into your body. So instead of just treating the symptom, you get to the root of your problem. The brain is not tricked into feeling any pain. Your pain actually goes away because the problem itself is resolved.

Inside your cells, you have a place where you store electrons/voltage called ATP. ATP is like the food of your cells and is like a rechargeable battery system. ATP is often referred to as the energy currency of life. If you want cash, you need an ATM machine, but if you want energy currency, you want ATP. Frequency specific microcurrent is like a battery charger with jumper cables connected to your cells. It restores your damaged cells to a healthy and vibrant electrical charge again.

Your body's cells use ATP to power almost all your activities, such as muscle contraction, protein construction, communication with your other cells and dismantling damaged and unused structures. Like a self-guided missile, FSM assists your body to achieve homeostasis, by correcting electrical abnormalities in your area of disease or injury.

Think of an Unhealthy Cell Like a Raisin and a Healthy and Vibrant Cell Like a Grape

RESTORE YOUR CELLS ELECTRICAL CHARGE AND RESTORE HEALTH AND VITALITY

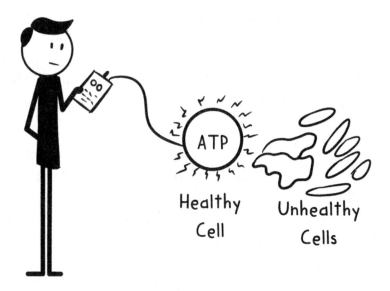

I have seen success using FSM with a broad range of acute and chronic conditions, including the following:

- Wound Healing
- Carpal Tunnel Syndrome
- Broken Bones

- Soft Tissue Regeneration
- Herpes/Shingles
- Chronic Fatigue
- Arthritis-Osteo and Rheumatoid
- Neurological Disorders
- Multiple Sclerosis
- Spinal Cord Injuries
- Plantar Fasciitis
- TMJ
- Neuropathy
- Nerve Entrapment
- Bell's Palsy
- Fibromyalgia
- Acute and Chronic Back Pain
- Headaches
- Disc Injuries/Tendonitis

What kind of results can I expect from these types of treatments?

Typical Patient Responses range from immediate and complete recovery in 3-5 sessions. In some cases, it may take 5-10 treatments before a breakthrough occurs. For severe cases, 12-15 treatments are more likely.

The effectiveness and sustainability of the treatments are always relative to the person and their commitment to supporting the healing process, which includes proper hydration along with a nutrition and lifestyle program.

Your Cellular Construction Crew

Let's visualize a construction crew building your new home. The workers are your cells that have specific jobs to do. The home they're building could be any injury or damaged/diseased tissue that you have in need of "rebuilding." What do the workers need to accomplish their task?

Let's review, they need three things:

1. Supplies - Supplies are your cells nutrition. Your cells build with nutrients, and each cell needs nutrients to work. The quality of the supplies directly affects the quality of the house. You wouldn't build a house with weak or rotted wood, and your cells can't build or repair your body with poor nutrients.

2. A clean working environment - to build a solid foundation, you would first remove the trees, shrubs, large rocks and other debris from the work area, creating a clean work environment. This waste represents the toxins in your body. You cannot build on the toxic or uneven soil.

3. Power - Finally, you need power. The workers' power tools run on batteries, which represent the batteries in each of your cells. If you don't have enough charge, the tools don't work, and the house can't be built.

A perfectly healthy body has the ability to naturally maintain a steady supply of "power" to its cells' batteries. However, most people are bombarded with numerous stressors from the modern world that prevent or block this natural flow of energy to the cells. Exposure to various stressors can all impact your body's capacity to renew its power.

Let's think about what would happen to this work crew if you cleared the land, gave them all the supplies they needed, such as blueprints, tools, and payment in full, but were unable to charge the batteries in their power tools? Not much work could be done. You'd have a crew with potential, but no power to cut wood, build a frame or put up walls.

This is the missing link in sick and injured people "cellular health," and FSM can bridge the gap.

FSM "recharges" your cells' batteries and with fully charged power tools and the right supplies, the crew is now ready to get to work.

Cellular health is the key to a pain-free, healthy and vibrant body and sometimes your body just needs a little help healing itself.

Chapter Nine

Are You Spending Enough Time with Dr. Happiness

We live in a complex world, but there are simple things we can do to be healthier, and one of those things is to make being happy a priority. Sometimes happiness can seem so elusive. We can convince ourselves into thinking we'd be happy if only—if only things were different, if only the world were different, if only we were different. We can convince ourselves that it's just a job away, or a relationship away, or a city away, only to get what we think we wanted and find ourselves still feeling unfulfilled.

At times, life can feel like a giant race with no finish line in sight. It can seem like we're always competing, striving, and struggling—pushing toward something better. Many of us learn from a young age that happiness is something we're entitled to pursue as if it's something we can chase, capture, and keep forever. It's this very thinking that makes it so challenging to feel joy and peace. We can't possibly experience happiness when we're worrying about making it last.

It's the tiny moment-to-moment choices we make that shape our experience of the world. We may not ever feel we have the perfect circumstances, but we can always choose to be mindful, grateful, optimistic, and open. Doing this simple thing can transform our perception.

One of the main things I love about my wife is her dedication to being happy. She loves to read positive, upbeat books, loves to be around happy and fun people and loves comedies! A pretty good strategy for being happy wouldn't you agree?

I think most people are about as happy as they make up their mind to be. Sometimes my wife has to remind me of this and thank goodness she does.

Did This Beatle Know the Key to Life?

I once read something about John Lennon and happiness that really brought a smile to my face. When John was a young boy, his mom told him happiness was the key to life. As part of an assignment at school, John's teacher had them write down what they wanted to be when they grew up? John wrote down "Happy" and the teacher said, "John I don't think you understand the assignment." and John looked at her and said, "I don't think you understand life."

I'm not sure if John Lennon actually ever said this because I couldn't find any anything concrete that backed this. However, I didn't really care cause it sounds cool and it made me happy just reading it.

The idea that you're either a glass-half-full person or a glass-half-empty person has almost begun to feel a little old-fashioned. Probably the most powerful message to arise from the new science of happiness is the idea that we can significantly change our outlook and life satisfaction no matter who we are, what we do, where we live or how much money we make.

"We are not our genes, our environments or our childhoods. At least, we don't have to be. By changing our habits, we can trump even our genes." We can all be glass-half-full people if we want.

- Start to make positive changes in your life like putting healthy foods in your body,
- Play music that inspires you or just that makes you feel good
- Be around nature, do anything that gets you outside
- Read books that inspire you.
- Watch movies that make you feel good because this actually releases endorphins that make you feel healthy
- Write what you are grateful for in a gratitude journal daily
- Be around water, showers, streams, oceans
- Do things that make you laugh and smile
- Watch comedies, listen to comedians and be around friends that make you laugh
- Do random acts of kindness
- Hold the door for strangers
- Smile at everyone
- Pick up garbage
- Text someone daily and ask how they are doing, show you care

Get in the "flow," and feel the satisfaction with your work, art or sport (by figuring out your core strengths and how you can best utilize them); meditate with Dr. Quiet; and exercise with Dr. Movement and eat well with Dr. Diet.

The way you think can transform the health of your body, and vice versa. You have a feedback loop that you can control and spin it in either direction you want. View stress as a challenge, not a threat.

By now you know that stress is bad for our health and emotional well-being. But worrying about whether you're too stressed can be stressful in itself. And who isn't juggling at least a half-dozen balls, none of which we can afford to drop? Stress-reduction strategies—meditation, massage, exercise, time with friends, etc.—are still great ideas, but some degree of stress will likely still be a part of your life no matter what. Find stress reduction strategies that work for you and quit trying to be perfect!

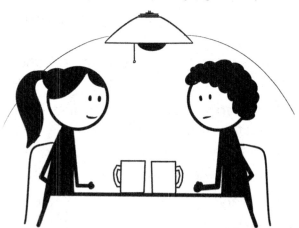

I WORK 12 HOURS A DAY, I EXERCISE 7 DAYS A WEEK,
I PREPARE HEALTHY MEALS AT HOME INSTEAD OF
GOING OUT AND IT'S ALL PAYING OFF. I'M FINALLY
TOO TIRED TO CARE ABOUT BEING PERFECT!

Think young

A new study actually shows you really are as young, and young-looking, as you think you are. Researchers from Harvard and M.I.T. examined how superficial cues of age (gray hair, baldness, etc.) affect health and longevity. Women were invited to a hair salon where they had their hair colored and/or cut. The women who thought their new 'dos made them look younger lowered their blood pressures, while those who didn't think the trip to the salon changed their appearance maintained the same blood pressure.

The lesson: Confidence in your appearance may actually make you better-looking.

Other examples of how the perception of age may speed up or slow down actual aging: Prematurely bald men are at greater risk of developing prostate cancer and coronary heart disease than men who aren't prematurely bald. The researchers guess, it is because the bald men perceive themselves as older. The point is not that baldness causes or is a precursor to cancer, but how you feel about it may play a part.

This same research found that women who have children late in life live longer than mothers who had their kids earlier, perhaps because they are surrounded by more signs of youth—infants, playgrounds, school, other (younger) parents—as they age. Another lesson: Play, swing and slide, and make friends of all ages.

Focus on the positives

Research has shown that if most of our interactions with others in a day are positive or neutral, and if one is negative, come bedtime, most of us will dwell on that one bad experience instead of focusing on the pleasant ones. This happens to most people even though the positive and neutral experiences were more frequent. It's a natural human psychological phenomenon called the "negativity bias": We give more weight to negative elements of our lives, and we spend more energy avoiding negative experiences than we do seeking positive ones. Even though I am generally a very positive person, I can get sucked into this as well.

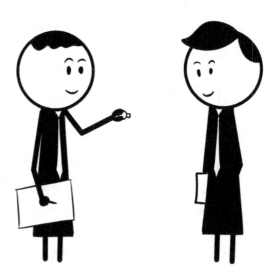

IT'S A SPECIAL HEARING AID. IT FILTERS OUT
CRITCSM AND AMPLIFIES COMPLIMENTS.

But what if we could reverse this? The mind-body connection is so strong that not only can we influence our health through our outlook—as demonstrated by the stress and hairstyle studies mentioned above. We can actually rewire our brains to respond and think in more productive ways. How? By "marinating in every good moment." Every time you have a pleasant experience, whether a hug from a friend or a family member, a joke shared in the elevator with a co-worker or running into an old friend on the street, savor the interaction afterward. Think about how it made you feel, why it was so great and how lucky you are to have such moments in your life.

Try to stay with this good moment for long enough - 12 or more seconds - so it transfers from short-term memory to long-term storage in your brain. Doing this a few times a day, you encourage a process that will gradually imprint these positive resources into your brain. In other words, chip away at your negativity focus until you can concentrate on the positive without effort.

Just as our neuroplasticity (the brain's ability to change) allows us to learn a new skill without thinking, we can train ourselves to think more positively. Before-and-after brain scans of people who practice this show physiological changes that reflect the shift away from the negativity focus.

Try not to focus on the past so much

Focused attention on bad feelings and experiences from the past—is a hallmark of depression. Reflection is a useless pattern of thinking that we all engage in, probably more than we should. When you're beating yourself up with questions like "Why did I ever do that?" or "How could I be so dumb?" you are "taking one more lap in hell," You may think you are gaining insight when you reflect, but what you're actually doing is re-triggering those negative emotions again and again and stimulating stress. Neurologically you are conditioning yourself to be afraid and to avoid those situations.

Instead, take it easy on yourself. So you had an embarrassing or humiliating moment. Acknowledge it and honor your feelings, learn what you can from it, and then move on. This is an area I personally still need to work on, but I am making progress.

Spend your money

Just do it wisely. It has been said that money can't buy happiness—at least once basic human needs are met. (One study found the cutoff to be $75,000; above that, more money didn't make a difference in personal well-being.) "Money is an opportunity for happiness, but it is an opportunity that people routinely squander because the things they think will make them happy often don't."

Studies have found that the money best spent is on experiences rather than material goods. (There! I just settled your vacation versus new-couch-and-TV dilemma.) Money also translates to happiness when it's spent on others rather than on you. (Doting grandmothers have known this for centuries.) Studies have actually shown that buying many small pleasures—a fancy chocolate truffle here, a new song on iTunes there—increases happiness more than splurging on a few large ones.

Find meaning

One of the biggest predictors of older people's health and life satisfaction, as they age, is their own self-reported sense of purpose in life. Possessing a strong sense of purpose was associated with increased ability to perform day-to-day activities and greater physical mobility. Seniors who had this strong sense of intention also had a lower risk of cognitive impairment and a slower rate of cognitive decline. They outlived their peers while enjoying a better quality of life.

Another recent study showed that having a deep sense of purpose allows faster and easier recovery from negative events.

Can you put others first? What is your social impact on the world? Living a life of purpose can be hard, and it has a long time frame when it comes to happiness. But in the end, it's the best measure of a happy life." Yes, meditate and find the flow and get coffee with friends and exercise and all those other proven positivity and health-enhancing boosters, but do so with a sense of purpose that makes them more than just feel-good activities. "That's the difference between a pleasant life and a truly happy one."

If you've been waiting for a meaningful life purpose to come to you, like a calling, you may want to go after it instead. Is it making the world better through your work or volunteerism? Is it taking care of your children and family? Is it creating art? Is it appreciating nature and helping with conservation efforts? Is it simply being an active and contributing member of your community?

Sing

While you're figuring out your purpose in life (no small task!), don't forget to sing. Many studies suggest that singing—with others, in a choir, by yourself, in the shower, or in the car along to the radio—releases a whole bunch of feel-good, pain-relieving, immunity-boosting chemicals in your body, including endorphins, serotonin, dopamine, and oxytocin. It has also been shown to lower cortisol, your stress hormone. Best part: The effects are the same whether you're in tune or not. Thank goodness for that!

Spend Time with Positive, Purpose Driven People

Find places and people that are supportive in helping you get better. Find people that share your same core values. Spend time with people that make you smile, laugh and feel good. And if you are ever given the assignment of writing down, what do you want to be when you grow up, just smile and write down, "Happy!"

In Conclusion

To really be as healthy, happy and fit as possible, make sure you invest time and energy into spending time with Dr. Diet, Dr. Quiet, Dr. Happiness and Dr. Movement. Find a team of holistic practitioners you can really trust to guide you on your health and fitness journey.

Here is what a great natural healer looks like:

They empathize with their client.

They always look for new ways to help their client improve.

They are never satisfied with their current level of results.

They expect what they recommend will work.

They are very hard on themselves if their treatment plan does not work as expected.

They communicate and collaborate with their team to ensure the best results for you.

They make you feel better just being around them.

Are you worth saving?

Imagine for a moment you are part of an emergency rescue team on a helicopter, and your job is to make a quick decision about whose life to save. A boat in the middle of the ocean has capsized, and there are four people in the water. You are low on fuel, and your rescue basket can hold only one person, so, unfortunately, you can only save one person. Who do you save?

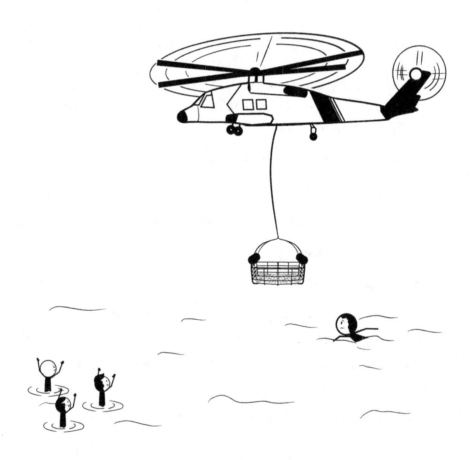

Rob J Smith

You save the person that is swimming towards you. If you want to feel, perform or look better so you can ultimately live better, then find "the right rescue basket" and swim like hell towards it. Your life just might depend on it!

Products and Services Rob Recommends

For helpful videos, tips and product and service recommendations by Rob and his wife Paula visit **www.AskRobandPaulaSmith.com.**

CPSIA information can be obtained
at www.ICGtesting.com
Printed in the USA
FSOW03n1120060118
42988FS

9 781641 366441